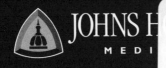

Patients' Guide to

Lung Cancer

Justin F. Klamerus, MD

Medical Oncology Fellow
Department of Oncology
The Sidney Kimmel Comprehensive Cancer Center at Johns Hopkins
Baltimore, MD

Julie R. Brahmer, MD, MSc

Assistant Professor of Oncology
Department of Oncology
The Sidney Kimmel Comprehensive Cancer Center at Johns Hopkins
Baltimore, MD

David S. Ettinger, MD, FACP, FCCP

Alex Grass Professor of Oncology
Department of Oncology
The Sidney Kimmel Comprehensive Cancer Center at Johns Hopkins
Baltimore, MD

SERIES EDITORS
Lillie D. Shockney, RN, BS, MAS

Administrative Director; Distinguished Service Associate Professor of Breast Cancer; Associate Professor,
Johns Hopkins University School of Medicine, Deptartments of Surgery and Gynecology; Associate
Professor, Johns Hopkins School of Nursing; Johns Hopkins Avon Foundation Breast Center
Baltimore, MD

Gary R. Shapiro, MD

Chairman, Department of Oncology
Johns Hopkins Bayview Medical Center
Director, Johns Hopkins Geriatric Oncology Program
The Sidney Kimmel Comprehensive Cancer Center at Johns Hopkins
Baltimore, MD

JONES & BARTLETT
L E A R N I N G

World Headquarters
Jones & Bartlett Learning
40 Tall Pine Drive
Sudbury, MA 01776
978-443-5000
info@jblearning.com
www.jblearning.com

Jones & Bartlett Learning
Canada
6339 Ormindale Way
Mississauga, Ontario L5V 1J2
Canada

Jones & Bartlett Learning
International
Barb House, Barb Mews
London W6 7PA
United Kingdom

Jones & Bartlett Learning books and products are available through most bookstores and online booksellers. To contact Jones & Bartlett Learning directly, call 800-832-0034, fax 978-443-8000, or visit our website, www.jblearning.com.

Substantial discounts on bulk quantities of Jones & Bartlett Learning publications are available to corporations, professional associations, and other qualified organizations. For details and specific discount information, contact the special sales department at Jones & Bartlett Learning via the above contact information or send an email to specialsales@jblearning.com.

The authors, editor, and publisher have made every effort to provide accurate information. However, they are not responsible for errors, omissions, or for any outcomes related to the use of the contents of this book and take no responsibility for the use of the products and procedures described. Treatments and side effects described in this book may not be applicable to all people; likewise, some people may require a dose or experience a side effect that is not described herein. Drugs and medical devices are discussed that may have limited availability controlled by the Food and Drug Administration (FDA) for use only in a research study or clinical trial. Research, clinical practice, and government regulations often change the accepted standard in this field. When consideration is being given to use of any drug in the clinical setting, the healthcare provider or reader is responsible for determining FDA status of the drug, reading the package insert, and reviewing prescribing information for the most up-to-date recommendations on dose, precautions, and contraindications, and determining the appropriate usage for the product. This is especially important in the case of drugs that are new or seldom used.

Production Credits
Executive Publisher: Christopher Davis
Editorial Assistant: Sara Cameron
Associate Production Editor: Laura Almozara
Associate Marketing Manager: Marion Kerr
V.P., Manufacturing and Inventory Control: Therese Connell
Composition: Appingo Publishing Services
Printing and Binding: Malloy, Inc.
Cover Design: Kristin E. Parker
Cover Image: © ImageZoo/age fotostock
Cover Printing: Malloy, Inc.

Library of Congress Cataloging-in-Publication Data

Klamerus, Justin.
  Johns Hopkins patients' guide to lung cancer / Justin Klamerus, Julie Brahmer, David Ettinger.
     p. cm. — (John Hopkins patients' guide)
  Includes bibliographical references and index.
  ISBN-13: 978-0-7637-7436-3
  ISBN-10: 0-7637-7436-7
  1. Lungs—Cancer. 2. Lungs—Cancer—Patients. 3. Lungs—Cancer—Treatment. I. Brahmer, Julie R. II. Ettinger, David S. III. Title.
  RC280.L8K53 2011
  616.99'462—dc22

                                        2009045694

6048

Printed in the United States of America
14 13 12 11 10   10 9 8 7 6 5 4 3 2 1

Dedication

This book is dedicated to our patients who have
been our principal teachers. Their courage inspires
all of us who have the privilege to care for patients
afflicted with cancer.

CONTENTS

CONTRIBUTORS' LIST

Lynn Billing, RN, CHPN
Nurse Coordinator
Harry J. Duffey Family Pain and Palliative Care Program
The Sidney Kimmel Comprehensive Cancer Center at
    Johns Hopkins
Baltimore, MD

Julie R. Brahmer, MD, MSc
Assistant Professor of Oncology, Department of Oncology
The Sidney Kimmel Comprehensive Cancer Center at
    Johns Hopkins
Baltimore, MD

Stephen Cattaneo, MD
Fellow, Department of Surgery
The Johns Hopkins Hospital
Baltimore, MD

Hongbin Chen, MD, PhD
Clinical Fellow, Department of Oncology
The Sidney Kimmel Comprehensive Cancer Center at
    Johns Hopkins
Baltimore, MD

Amy E. DeZern, MD
ACS Instructor, Department of Medicine
The Johns Hopkins Hospital
Baltimore, MD

David S. Ettinger, MD, FACP, FCCP
Alex Grass Professor of Oncology, Department
    of Oncology
The Sidney Kimmel Compehensive Cancer Center at
    Johns Hopkins
Baltimore, MD

Russell Hales, MD
Resident, Department of Radiation Oncology and
    Molecular Radiation Sciences
The Sidney Kimmel Comprehensive Cancer Center at
    Johns Hopkins
Baltimore, MD

Christine Hann, MD, PhD
Assistant Professor of Oncology, Department of Oncology
The Sidney Kimmel Comprehensive Cancer Center at
    Johns Hopkins
Baltimore, MD

Mary M. Hesdorffer, CRNP
Nurse Practitioner, Department of Oncology
The Sidney Kimmel Comprehensive Cancer Center at
    Johns Hopkins
Baltimore, MD

Rosalyn Juergens, MD
Assistant Professor of Oncology, Department of Oncology
The Sidney Kimmel Comprehensive Cancer Center at
    Johns Hopkins
Baltimore, MD

Justin F. Klamerus, MD
Medical Oncology Fellow, Department of Oncology
The Sidney Kimmel Comprehensive Cancer Center at
   Johns Hopkins
Baltimore, MD

Donald List, MSW, LCSW-C
Senior Clinical Social Worker
Patient Family Services and Oncology Social Work
The Sidney Kimmel Comprehensive Cancer Center at
   Johns Hopkins
Baltimore, MD

Carole Seddon, MA, LCSW-C, BCD, OSW-C
Senior Clinical Social Worker
Patient Family Services and Oncology Social Work
The Sidney Kimmel Comprehensive Cancer Center at
   Johns Hopkins
Baltimore, MD

Teresa Seeger, CRNP
Nurse Practitioner, Department of Oncology
The Sidney Kimmel Compehensive Cancer Center at
   Johns Hopkins
Baltimore, MD

Gary R. Shapiro, MD
Chairman, Department of Oncology
Visiting Associate, Department of Oncology
Director, Johns Hopkins Geriatric Oncology Program
Johns Hopkins Bayview Medical Center
Baltimore, MD

Danny Song, MD
Assistant Professor of Radiation Oncology and Molecular
  Radiation Sciences
Department of Radiation Oncology and Molecular
  Radiation Sciences
The Sidney Kimmel Comprehensive Cancer Center at
  Johns Hopkins
Baltimore, MD

Cynthia Williams, DO, MA
Palliative Care Physician
Harry J. Duffey Family Pain and Palliative Care Program
The Sidney Kimmel Comprehensive Cancer Center at
  Johns Hopkins
Baltimore, MD

PREFACE

Lung cancer is a common illness, and being diagnosed with it makes you a member of a large and growing community. There are over 200,000 newly diagnosed cases in the United States every year. Lung cancer is the leading cause of cancer mortality in both men and women in the United States and worldwide.

Despite these sobering statistics, this is a time of increasing hope and excitement in the lung cancer community. Several new therapies have emerged in the past few years, leading to progressive improvements in both survival and quality of life for people with lung cancer. Among the most notable milestones marking progress are studies showing that chemotherapy improves chance of survival for patients with surgically resected lung cancer, and that novel "targeted" therapies improve survival in patients with unresectable and even recurrent lung cancer. There have been major improvements in radiation and surgical approaches, leading to fewer side effects and better outcomes. There have been great strides in supportive care measures, perhaps most notably the introduction of much more effective antinausea medications. Research in lung cancer is beginning to change the poor prognosis of this disease, and new approaches are being tested every week in our clinics.

This book is intended to serve as an introduction to the diagnosis of lung cancer, written for our patients, their families, and friends. Our goals in preparing this volume are to try to provide a better understanding of the disease and how it may be treated, what to expect during treatment, and, importantly, what to expect after treatment. The physical and emotional stresses of this illness and the impact of its sometimes aggressive therapies are an increasing focus of attention as the lung cancer survivorship community grows.

One of the most important aspects of lung cancer treatment in the 21st century is the team, or multidisciplinary, approach. The newly diagnosed patient quickly becomes the central member of a large team, including professionals from various walks of life who work together to define the right therapy options for this particular individual at this particular time. The authorship of this book reflects the diversity of that team, drawing from the many disciplines that comprise our lung cancer program at Johns Hopkins.

I hope that this book may serve as a guide to understanding the roles of the various members of your team, what their expertise may be, and what they have to offer in supporting you through your cancer treatment. Reading may prompt more questions than answers. All questions are good questions! I encourage you to write them down, and use this as a starting point for conversations with your healthcare providers about your options.

I hope that you find this book helpful.

Charles M. Rudin, MD, PhD
Associate Director for Clinical Research
Director of Lung Cancer Therapeutics
Co-Director of the Upper Aerodigestive Cancer Program
The Sidney Kimmel Comprehensive Cancer Center
at Johns Hopkins
Baltimore, MD

Acknowledgments

Sincerest gratitude to Evan and Carol Davis for their generous contribution to the production of this book. Their love and support will always be treasured.

Justin F. Klamerus

INTRODUCTION

HOW TO USE THIS BOOK
TO YOUR BENEFIT

The goal of this book is to help you learn more about your cancer and make informed decisions about your care. By being better informed, we hope you will be better prepared to confront the challenges ahead as you proceed through treatment and recovery. You will receive a lot of information from your healthcare team and will probably search the Internet or bookstores. No doubt friends and family members who mean well will attempt to give you advice about what to do and when to do it and will try to steer you in certain directions.

Yes, your doctor has told you that you have lung cancer. Although the diagnosis of lung cancer is frightening, there is hope. Hearing the diagnosis is difficult, but with support and accurate information to make good decisions, you can participate in decision-making about your care and treatment.

This book is designed to be a guide that takes you through the various treatment options and side effects and will help you put together a plan of action so that you become a lung cancer survivor. The book contains information about current surgical, radiotherapeutic, and systemic (i.e., chemotherapy, targeted therapy) therapeutic options; and combined modality treatment options; as well as recommendations for living with and surviving cancer. There is also a glossary in the back and resources listed for your further review and information. This information will help you to understand the how, when, and why of treatment options.

Let's begin now with the understanding of what has happened and what the first steps are to get you well again.

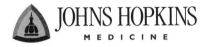

FIRST STEPS—
I'VE BEEN DIAGNOSED
WITH LUNG CANCER

JUSTIN F. KLAMERUS, MD; AND
DAVID S. ETTINGER, MD, FACP, FCCP

There is perhaps no greater life-altering moment than when you or a loved one has been diagnosed with cancer. The first time patients hear this news from their doctors, they often describe being frozen in time and unable to remember much of this initial conversation. Many emotions surround this time and each individual and his or her loved ones will have unique and widely varied responses. Avoidance might be the natural response to your new diagnosis—the feeling that if only you could run away and go back to the time before your diagnosis was made, all would be well again. Or you might respond in a much more assertive manner and believe that if you can assemble all of the right resources, no hurdle is insurmountable. There is no right response. Each person's journey through cancer will be unlike any other. The work of those of us who care for patients afflicted with cancer, both personally and professionally, is to be a source of comfort and reassurance. Our goal: No one who faces cancer will face cancer alone!

This book will serve as a field guide to navigating lung cancer. We hope that each chapter will help to prepare patients and their loved ones to be well informed and prepared for the road ahead. Former Surgeon General Dr. C. Everett Koop once said, "The best prescription is knowledge." We believe this to be true as well and hope to accompany you through the process of adjustment, acceptance, understanding, and action.

DIAGNOSIS AND PROGNOSIS

We begin with the diagnosis. Cancer is a commonly used term and you are probably already familiar with the meaning. Medically speaking, cancer is a broad term used to describe cells that have escaped the body's methods to control growth and reproduction. This uncontrolled growth can lead cells that arise in one location to grow into tumors that may spread and grow in other locations in the body. When cancer has spread it is called metastasis.

Cancers are widely variable diseases and the organ in which they develop often indicates how aggressive they are. Lung cancer is a serious disease. The condition is slightly more prevalent in men than women; however, lung cancer is the second most common cancer in both men and women in the United States. Although the average age at diagnosis is 71, lung cancer can develop at any age. One reality that is particularly distressing for patients and their loved ones is the statistics related to lung cancer survival. Unfortunately, lung cancer remains the leading cause of cancer death in the world. More patients die each year from lung cancer than from breast, colon, and prostate cancer combined.

Despite these very real challenges, much progress has been made through research in the last decade. Not only are more therapies available to treat the disease, many of these therapies are considered "targeted," with special design to attack unique functions that tumors use to grow. These novel forms of therapy have different side effect profiles, and these, along with improved supportive care, make lung cancer treatment today much different than it was 5 or 10 years ago.

LEARNING ABOUT YOUR DISEASE

Lung cancer is a very broad diagnosis that encompasses cancers that arise within the airways or lungs. It is categorized into two major types: non-small cell lung cancer (NSCLC) and small cell lung cancer (SCLC) (see Table 1). The complexity doesn't stop there. The lung cancers are further divided into various subtypes, which are determined by how these cancers look under the microscope. Your physicians will rely on the detailed biopsy reports from pathologists to determine the type of lung cancer you or your loved one has been diagnosed with.

The type of lung cancer, together with the stage of disease, dictates the treatment approach. In general, patients diagnosed with SCLC receive chemotherapy and/or radiation therapy as the main forms of therapy, while patients with NSCLC can be treated with surgery, chemotherapy, and/ or radiation therapy. See Chapter 3 for more information about treatment.

3

Table 1 Types of Lung Cancer

Types	Sub-types
Non-Small Cell Lung Cancer *85% of cases*	• Adenocarcinomas (50–60% of NSCLC) • Squamous Cell Carcinomas (20–25% of NSCLC) • Large Cell Carcinomas (15% of NSCLC) • Uncommon: Neuroendocrine or Carcinoid Tumors, Carcinosarcomas, Cystic Adenoid Carcinomas
Small Cell Lung Cancer *15% of cases*	• Oat Cell (lymphocyte-like) • Polygonal Cell • Fusiform • Mixed

In cancer medicine, the key factors your doctors will use to determine your treatment plan are:

1. What type of lung cancer has been diagnosed?

2. How advanced is the cancer (localized or metastatic)?

3. What is the general health status of the patient and are some forms of treatment too hazardous?

These factors are explored in later sections of the book.

RISK FACTORS

There are many known risk factors for developing lung cancer; however, the most significant risk comes from cigarette smoking. Smoking is responsible for approximately 87% of cases of lung cancer. Other risk factors include: exposure to second-hand or passive smoke, radon gas (decay product from uranium and radium), asbestos, and smoke from burning wood; and certain forms of benign lung diseases (interstitial fibrosis, asbestosis, and chronic obstructive pulmonary disease, or COPD). Patients and their families are often concerned about the genetic risks of lung cancer. Although no single gene has been identified, there is a small increased risk of first-degree relatives developing lung cancer when another family member has been affected. This risk increases if the affected family member's lung cancer was diagnosed at an early age or if lung cancer has affected many members of the family.

Although most patients who develop lung cancer are current or former smokers, lung cancer can develop in patients with little or no significant past history of smoking. One alarming statistic is the increasing number of cases that occur in patients who have never smoked. Approximately 1 out of 5 women who develop lung cancer has never been a smokers and 1 out of 10 men has never been a smoker. Much research is being directed at patients with limited smoking histories because some forms of treatment seem to work better in patients who were light smokers or who never smoked.

UNDERSTANDING HOW YOUR LUNG CANCER IS STAGED

Cancer staging systems have been established to standardize treatment plans and to help physicians make predictions about a patient's prognosis. In general, the lower the stage, the better the prognosis. One system, proposed by the American Joint Committee on Cancer (AJCC), assesses the size of the tumor (T), the presence or absence of involved lymph nodes (N), and existence of metastasis (M) to define the stage of cancer for each patient. The stage of cancer is usually written as roman numerals I–IV. This staging system is commonly used for NSCLC and is particularly complex. It is based on whether the tumor is big or small; whether it invades nearby structures; whether the regional lymph nodes are involved on the same side or opposite side of the tumor, or have tumor in the lymph nodes located under the breast bone; whether there is a great deal of tumor in the lymph nodes or only a microscopic amount of disease; and lastly whether there is distant metastatic disease. We recommend that you discuss the factors involved in staging your cancer with your oncologist.

Patients with early stage lung cancer (stages I–II) are usually able to undergo surgical resection and have a better chance of survival. Stage IV NSCLC, the most advanced stage, is defined as cancer that has spread to a distant site (metastatic cancer) and for which surgical removal offers the patient no survival benefit. Stage III cancers are in the middle. This stage is divided into stage IIIA and IIIB disease. Stage III lung cancers are cancers that have not spread to other organs beyond the lymph nodes of the chest. If you have been diagnosed with a stage III cancer, please ask your surgeon and oncologist to describe the key differences between stage IIIA and IIIB cancers. Treatment for these two stages is distinctly different.

For SCLC, a two-stage system is most often used—"limited stage" or "extensive stage." Limited stage usually indicates that the cancer is "limited" to one lung, and if lymph nodes are involved, these lymph nodes are on the same side of the chest as the primary tumor. Extensive stage SCLC usually exists when the cancer has spread (metastasized) to distant sites. For more information on lung cancer staging and the procedures used for it, see Chapter 2.

HOW TO SELECT YOUR ONCOLOGY TEAM AND CANCER CENTER

As you move along in your understanding of this disease, a key decision early in the course of the diagnosis is the selection of your treatment team. Chapter 2 will describe in detail each of the members of this team—medical oncologists, radiation oncologists, thoracic surgeons, nurses, and other specialists who will help to coordinate treatment.

First and foremost, you must make sure that your oncologist is competent and knowledgeable about the treatment of your particular type of lung cancer. In general, lung cancer is a disease that many medical oncologists are comfortable treating. As cancers go, it is a relatively common disease and as such, most oncologists have treated many patients with lung cancer. Still, it is a good idea to ask your primary care physician and any other doctors who may refer you to suggest oncologists who have experience or interest in treating lung cancer.

The American Board of Internal Medicine is a professional organization that oversees the skills and knowledge necessary to become "Board Certified" in a medical specialty. We recommend that whomever you or your loved one choose for an oncologist, that she/he be "Board Certified" in medical oncology. Upon request, your oncologist's office should be very willing to share this information with you. The American Society of Clinical Oncology has an excellent Web site for patients and their families at http://www.asco.org/portal/site/patient. In particular, the "Find an Oncologist" quick link might be particularly helpful with this step in your journey.

In addition to the knowledge and understanding needed to provide patients with the most up-to-date treatment, oncologists also should be compassionate and empathic. Patients often say that they don't care how much their doctors know until they know how much their doctors care. Finding a caring and compassionate oncologist is critical for the type of doctor–patient relationship that is needed for patients who face cancer. Most physicians enter medicine because they wish to ease suffering; in oncology, this altruism runs high. Still, many doctors face pressures that limit the time they have to be a source of support and compassion for their patients. Patient volume, insurance red tape, and many other factors push and pull your healthcare providers and take them away from their most rewarding work. We recommend asking in advance how much time you will be given for initial and subsequent visits with your oncologist. Whenever possible, it is also helpful to ask friends and family, community members, or local cancer support groups who may have direct experience with your oncologist to give their opinions of your prospective oncologist.

Along with the individual choice of your oncologist, you must also decide what type of medical practice setting in which you would like to be treated. Whenever possible, we encourage you to seek out an accredited (i.e., American College of Surgeons or National Cancer Institute) cancer center with a lung cancer program. These centers are focused specifically on treating cancer patients and all of their resources and expertise will be directed to malignant diseases.

GATHERING RECORDS

Before your first visit at the cancer center, it is very helpful to have assembled all relevant medical records. Your cancer specialist will want to review all of your records, and you should bring them with you to your first visit. You may need to sign an "Authorization for Release of Information" before these records are released, and you can do this in person, through the mail, or by fax. You might now be thinking, "Why do I need to do all of this? Why do I have to get these documents or reports?" Accredited cancer centers are required to re-examine the images, and the pathology slides in particular, to verify their accuracy. There are situations in which a repeat evaluation by a pathologist could reveal an error or modify the diagnosis. Correct information ultimately helps your surgeon or oncologist determine the best plan of care for you.

The accuracy of your diagnosis is extremely important. Even if you have been told that you have a particular form of lung cancer, a second opinion from another pathologist may be requested because accurate diagnosis is crucial for successful treatment. Moreover, it is not enough to say you have lung cancer. Is it non-small or small cell lung cancer? If you have non-small cell lung cancer, what is the subtype? Is it adenocarcinoma, squamous cell carcinoma, or large cell carcinoma? Therapy is dependent on this information.

We recommend that you bring the following:

- Biopsy reports and the actual pathology slides.
- Digitized computed tomography (CT) scans, magnetic resonance imaging (MRI), or X-rays that are burned to a CD. If this isn't possible, the actual films are also fine.
- Laboratory test results.
- Recent pulmonary function tests (PFTs), if available.
- Copies of operative reports, if applicable.

- Copies of notes or letters from consulting doctors.

- A summary of your past medical history, including any chronic conditions or significant illnesses.

- A list of all of the medications you are taking, with strengths and dosage schedules.

Once these records are gathered, it is important to have these available at all visits, especially when seeing providers for the first time. As treatment progresses, it is a good idea to keep these health records accurate and up to date. Many of the therapies used to treat cancer may be unfamiliar to doctors who don't specialize in cancer medicine. In addition to the above, we suggest including the following information:

- A record of all surgeries you have had, with dates of procedures and the names of all surgeons

- A summary of all chemotherapy agents you have received, including dates, and a record of side effects

- A summary report describing any radiation therapy you have received, if applicable

- A list of your treating physicians, with important contact numbers

There are many resources available to help you and your family understand and cope with a lung cancer diagnosis. We hope that this book, including the trusted resources presented in Chapter 11, will be a helpful resource for you. Now that we have provided an initial foundation, let's move on and introduce the doctors, nurses, and allied professionals who will form your treatment team.

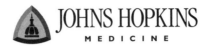

CHAPTER 2

MY TEAM— MEETING YOUR TREATMENT TEAM

MARY M. HESDORFFER, CRNP; JUSTIN F. KLAMERUS, MD; AND DAVID S. ETTINGER, MD, FACP, FCCP

The title of this chapter is very appropriate to the practice of medicine today. You are considered the most valuable member of the team and your input is extremely important to the medical staff. Your treatment team will be made up of multiple doctors and specialists who will work together. Each has a specific role in your treatment, and the following is a list of the major players, along with their descriptions:

> *Medical Oncologist.* This is a physician who has completed advanced training in cancer medicine and specializes in diagnosing and treating cancer using chemotherapy, hormonal therapy, and biological therapy. The selection of the medical oncologist is a particularly important decision because this physician will function as the team leader for most patients, coordinating testing and care among team members.

Surgical Oncologist. A surgeon with advanced training in cancer surgery.

Radiation Oncologist. A medical doctor who is trained to use radiation to treat cancer. Many but not all forms of cancer are treated with radiation therapy.

Radiologist. This is a medical doctor who obtains special training in the interpretation of tests such as X-rays and CT scans. The radiologist plays a crucial role in helping your physicians and surgeons to plan their approach to your cancer.

Pathologist. This is a medical doctor trained in the diagnosis of disease by studying cells and tissues under a microscope. Your pathologist will study your biopsy to determine the size of your tumor.

Pulmonologist. This is a medical doctor specializing in diseases of the lung.

Thoracic Surgeon. This is a surgeon who specializes in surgical management of diseases of the chest. The thoracic surgeon can determine the stage of your cancer by removing and studying a portion of your lung that includes the tumor and associated lymph nodes. In addition to obtaining tissue for the diagnostic biopsy, the thoracic surgeon often removes a portion of the lung, including the lung tumor and associated lymph nodes, to determine the ultimate stage of the cancer.

Physicians Assistants and Nurse Practitioners. These team members have advanced training to examine patients and write prescriptions as well as an in-depth understanding of lung cancer and its treatments. They will work closely with your specialist physicians and surgeons, and are under their direct supervision. In addition, most of the nurses you will encounter have specialty training and experience in their discipline of oncology. Quietly working in the background will be a group of highly specialized pharmacists who will monitor your routine medications and chemotherapy while diligently checking for dose accuracy and medication interactions.

Social Worker. An oncology social worker provides counseling, education, information, and referrals to community resources to people with cancer. They can help the patient and their family navigate the healthcare environment as well as help them manage the day-to-day challenges of living with cancer.

Survivor Volunteer. A lung cancer survivor who is interested in assisting lung cancer patients, provides emotional support throughout the treatment process – as well as beyond if the patient desires.

PREPARING FOR YOUR FIRST VISIT

Once you have selected your oncologist, it is important to be as prepared as possible for your first visit. Bring a small but supportive group of family or friends. Having a large number of people with you can be overpowering and, in our experience, prevents the patient from having all of his or her issues attended to. Write out a list of your questions for the oncologist and give copies of the list to a family member or friend so that he/she can help to make sure that all of the questions are answered. A list of good questions to ask follows:

1. What type of lung cancer do I have?

2. Did you feel anything abnormal when you examined me?

3. What stage of disease do you think I have based on what you know so far from my clinical examination, imaging studies, and tests?

4. Am I a candidate for surgery? How did you make this determination?

5. Did your pathology team confirm the accuracy of the biopsy results?

6. How soon will my surgery be scheduled?

7. What educational information do you offer to prepare me for surgery and what to expect?

8. Who will be my contact here for questions I may have?

9. Do you have educational materials for other family members?

10. How many lung cancer surgeries do you perform a year?

11. How long have you been in practice doing lung cancer surgeries?

12. Who else will be involved in my care, and when will I meet them?

13. How soon after surgery will I see a medical oncologist and/or radiation oncologist if needed?

14. Do you anticipate I will need chemotherapy, and if so, why?

15. Do you anticipate I will need radiation, and if so, why?

16. How often will I be seeing you for ongoing evaluation after my surgery?

17. Who will be coordinating my care?

18. How are subsequent appointments arranged for me, and when do these happen?

Some of those questions are better suited for different oncology specialists, such as your medical oncologist, thoracic surgeon, etc.

WHAT TO BRING WITH YOU TO YOUR APPOINTMENTS

Once you have made the necessary appointments, remember to bring a notebook with you to your doctor visits. In the notebook, record important information, concerns that you have and important names and numbers. Along with your notebook, be sure to bring a calendar with you. You will be given many appointments and it can be quite overwhelming if you do not have a system to keep track of these dates. With a notebook and calendar in hand, you can also discuss your schedule with the specialists, as well as plan family and social events around this busy time. It is important that all cancer patients enjoy time with family and friends. Be sure to tell your healthcare team about important events so that your treatment plan can accommodate these special times. If timing of a test or treatment is critical, your doctors will not compromise your care by adjusting the schedule; however, in most cases there is great flexibility in the timing of procedures and therapy.

DETERMINING YOUR CANCER'S STAGE

STAGING

One of the first steps in the process of determining an individual's plan of care is to determine the extent of cancer within the patient's body, which is done by performing diagnostic radiographic tests. CT scans evaluate the size, location, and possible spread of tumor with more clarity and detail than regular X-rays. CT imaging combines special X-ray equipment with sophisticated computers to produce multiple images or pictures of the inside of the body. These images can then be examined on a computer monitor. Because a CT scan requires dye that might be damaging to the kidneys, blood tests (creatinine) are ordered to make sure that your kidneys are healthy enough to eliminate this dye. Be sure to let your doctor know if you have a history of an allergy to contrast dye. You may need to have a CT scan without dye or get premedicated to prevent a serious allergic reaction. CT scans of the abdomen and pelvis also require you to fast for at least 6 hours and drink a contrast liquid shortly before the scan.

CT images of the chest and abdomen help determine the cancer's stage. Many patients also get a PET (positive emissions tomography) scan to further clarify the extent of the cancer. Unlike other scanning techniques, a PET scan isn't designed to show the structural detail of organs; instead, it tests for metabolic activity within certain organs or tissues. This metabolic activity often correlates with the presence of cancerous cells, and a PET scan may detect cancers in areas of the body that were missed by more traditional scanning methods. Because high blood sugar levels can render the test inaccurate, you will need to fast overnight before the scan. If you are diabetic, please request special instructions from your imaging center prior to the PET scan. Many institutions have the ability to combine both the CT scan and PET scan in one machine, which is known as a CT/PET.

Lung cancer can sometimes spread to the brain, so it is customary to obtain either a CT scan with intravenous contrast or an MRI of the brain as part of initial staging evaluation.

Unlike X-rays or CT scans, which use radiation, MRI uses powerful magnets and radio waves. You will be asked to lie very still during this procedure and you will hear very loud noises as the magnets are raised and lowered. If you have difficulty lying still for extended periods of time or suffer from claustrophobia or anxiety, inform your doctor so that he or she can prescribe a medication to help you relax during this procedure.

After your staging imaging studies have been completed, it often takes a few days for the official results to be made available. The results will be issued to your doctors, but we encourage you to obtain copies of these diagnostic study reports for your own personal records.

BIOPSY

A sample of your tumor must be obtained to correctly identify what type of lung cancer you have. This is called a biopsy. Before you have a biopsy, the physician responsible for performing the procedure will meet with you to explain its risks and benefits, as well as any alternatives to the particular procedure. Be sure to tell your doctor all of your current medications, including over-the-counter preparations, and avoid aspirin and ibuprofen prior to the procedure since they can cause excessive bleeding. You should ask your doctor when you can resume taking these medications.

When the primary lung tumor is located in the center of the chest close to one of the large air tubes, it is usually possible to use a bronchoscope to do the biopsy. A bronchoscope allows the pulmonologist or thoracic surgeon to visualize your lungs. There are two types of bronchoscopes: flexible and rigid. The rigid bronchoscope requires that you be asleep under general anesthesia in the operating room. Since the flexible bronchoscope can be used in the outpatient setting while you are getting intravenous medicines to help you relax and feel drowsy, it is used more often than the rigid bronchoscope. Most patients are somewhat sleepy after this procedure, so be sure to have someone accompany you to the hospital on the day of your bronchoscopy.

During the bronchoscopy, the airways are visualized and concerning areas biopsied and evaluated for the presence of cancer. The bronchoscope is inserted into the patient's trachea, or windpipe, to the location of the suspected tumor. Needle biopsies of lymph nodes around the trachea can then be performed during the procedure depending on their size and location. Most patients will be discharged home following a short recovery period.

Tumors that are not close to a bronchus are hard to reach with a bronchoscope, and, if the CT scan shows your tumor is one of these, your biopsy will probably be done by passing a needle through the skin into the tumor (percutaneous needle biopsy). This procedure is done by an interventional radiologist who uses a CT scanner to pinpoint the exact location of the tumor in your body. During this procedure, the radiologist uses a very thin needle and syringe to withdraw tissue or fluid specimens from an organ or suspected tumor mass while it is being viewed on a CT scan. You must be able to lie flat and very still in order to perform a CT-guided percutaneous needle biopsy, and since many lung cancer patients find this difficult, it is important that you make your physicians aware of any concerns that you may have.

There is little pain involved with this outpatient procedure and it usually takes only 30 minutes to complete. An X-ray of your lungs is usually obtained following this procedure to monitor for any complications from the biopsy.

Sometimes neither a bronchoscopy nor percutaneous needle biopsy can be done, and it is necessary for a surgeon to do the biopsy in the operating room. There are a number of techniques available to surgeons, and these are discussed in Chapter 3.

MEDIASTINOSCOPY

A mediastinoscopy is a procedure that is performed by a thoracic surgeon primarily to evaluate the lymph nodes surrounding the windpipe. In many circumstances, if these lymph nodes contain cancer cells, surgery is delayed until after chemotherapy and radiation are given. General anesthesia is used for this procedure with patients completely asleep in the operating room. A small cut is made over the windpipe just above the breastbone. A scope is advanced through the incision, allowing the surgeon to view the entire outside of the windpipe and any enlarged lymph nodes located in this region of the chest called the mediastinum. The major risk of this procedure is bleeding, as major blood vessels to the head and arms are located nearby within this space. Fortunately, major bleeding is very uncommon. Similar to bronchoscopy, following a brief recovery, most patients go home the same day.

MULTIDISCIPLINARY TUMOR BOARD

Once the results of your scans and biopsy are available, your case may be discussed at a special meeting of doctors and health professionals called a "Tumor Board." This is a special multidisciplinary meeting where pulmonologists, radiologists, surgeons, medical oncologists, radiation oncologists, and pathologists all get together to determine the best possible treatment for patients diagnosed with cancer.

PALLIATIVE CARE

One specialty in oncology that is often underutilized by physicians and patients is palliative care. Professionals (doctors, nurses, PAs/NPs, pharmacists, social workers, psychologists, chaplains) involved in palliative medicine focus on the palliation, or relief, of the symptoms associated with cancer, and they are an important contributor to the multidisciplinary tumor board. More information on this form of care is provided in Chapter 9. In order to better understand what services can be provided to help you with your symptoms, we encourage you to consult with the palliative care professionals available at your treatment center.

FINANCIAL IMPLICATIONS OF TREATMENT AND INSURANCE CLEARANCE

If you are experiencing financial problems or just having difficulty coping with your disease, an oncology social worker can be an invaluable resource and many cancer treatment centers have these personnel available to assist you. If you have family members or friends willing to assist, assign one person to keep track of insurance and medical bills. This will enable you to focus on your treatment plan without the distractions and stress of record keeping.

Prior to scheduling visits with your doctors, it is important to verify that these providers accept your insurance. Occasionally, some insurance plans will require a referral to see specialists, like oncologists and surgical oncologists. It is your responsibility to obtain all necessary referrals from your primary care physician. Cancer is a complex disease and requires multiple specialists. It can be very helpful to ask your insurer to provide you with a case manager who is an individual assigned to manage your insurance needs and who will be a contact for your doctor's office staff as well. If any form of your treatment is denied, this individual will assist you in an appeals process and can facilitate a quick turnaround.

Treating cancer is a complex and individualized process and all patients should utilize the skill and expertise of the entire team to receive the best treatment possible. The next chapter will focus on the various treatment options that are available to patients diagnosed with lung cancer.

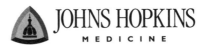

TAKING ACTION— COMPREHENSIVE TREATMENT CONSIDERATIONS

STEPHEN CATTANEO, MD; JUSTIN F. KLAMERUS, MD; RUSSELL HALES, MD; DANNY SONG, MD; AND ROSALYN JUERGENS, MD

The treatment of lung cancer is complex. As Chapter 2 introduced, there are many different kinds of specialists involved in the treatment of lung cancer. Chapter 3 will serve as an important reference for three key components of lung cancer treatment—surgery, radiation, and chemotherapy. Not all patients receive each form of therapy as these decisions are highly individualized to each patient.

SECTION 1: SURGERY
STEPHEN CATTANEO, MD; AND JUSTIN F. KLAMERUS, MD

OVERVIEW

As discussed in Chapter 2, sometimes a surgical procedure is necessary to establish the diagnosis of lung cancer. In addition to obtaining tissue for the diagnostic biopsy, the thoracic surgeon often removes a portion of the lung, including the lung tumor and associated lymph nodes, to determine the ultimate stage of the cancer. Depending upon the patient's stage of cancer, the surgeon may remove the entire tumor or perform other surgical procedures to assist with palliation of symptoms.

STAGING

In order to diagnose a lung nodule or mass as cancer, a portion of the tissue needs to be collected and sent for evaluation by a pathologist. Often times this can be performed by using a CT-guided needle biopsy or during a specialized procedure called a bronchoscopy, which is typically performed by a pulmonologist or thoracic surgeon. The procedure involves inserting a small camera down inside a patient's trachea, or windpipe, to the location of the suspected tumor. A biopsy can then be performed with a small needle attached to the camera.

For some patients, a more involved surgical procedure will be necessary to diagnose a lung cancer. For example, a tumor may be in a location within the lung that is not accessible by a needle, or the small amount of tissue obtained by the needle biopsy may have been insufficient to determine the diagnosis. Typically this is done by a wedge excision of the suspected cancer. A wedge excision is a surgical procedure in which a tumor is removed along with a portion of normal lung. An additional component of surgical staging may involve an assessment of the lymph nodes around the trachea. If lymph nodes are enlarged or demonstrate increased activity by CT and/or PET imaging, a mediastinoscopy may be performed by the thoracic surgeon. This is a special procedure in which the surgeon inserts a camera into the space in the chest that separates the two lungs. This procedure is described in more detail below.

TUMOR REMOVAL

Pulmonary function tests (PFTs) should be performed prior to undergoing a surgical procedure. PFTs allow for an overall assessment of a patient's ability to breathe and help predict the amount of lung that can be safely removed during surgery. If too much lung is removed, patients may have significant impairment in their ability to breathe normally. In some cases, PFTs will help your physicians to predict if you will need supplemental oxygen therapy following surgery. For some patients, the size of the tumor and the health of the lungs may prevent the thoracic surgeon from removing the tumor. One special test, called a ventilation-perfusion (V/Q) scan, may be ordered to gain further information as to the health of a particular region of the lung. The V/Q scan helps determine what fraction of your pulmonary function is from the portion of the lung to be removed. This test is often performed to help your doctors understand if a patient is a good candidate for surgical removal of the tumor.

Following these tests, a surgeon will need to perform a thorough clinical assessment of candidates for surgery. All of the test results will be reviewed by a surgeon so that he or she can plan the type of surgical procedure to be performed. At times a balance between the ideal cancer operation and a patient's ability to tolerate lung tissue removal must be found so that adequate recovery from the operation is possible. The diagnostic tests described above along with any surgeries performed will help the surgeon and pathologist to stage the patient's lung cancer. If surgery is an option for you or your loved one, several types of operations can be performed to remove the tumor and reduce the risk that the tumor grows back following surgery. The choice of procedure will depend on where the tumor is located, the number of lesions, and the medical condition of the patient.

TYPES OF LUNG CANCER SURGERIES

The following operations are used to treat lung cancer:

1. Wedge excision or segmentectomy

2. Lobectomy

3. Pneumonectomy

If the thoracic surgeon removes the cancerous lesion and a small amount of normal lung surrounding the tumor, the operation is called a wedge excision. A wedge excision is done if the tumor is in a location in the lung that is not accessible by a needle. If a larger amount of surrounding normal lung is removed, the surgery is called a segmentectomy. In this operation, an entire segment of the lung is removed. Wedge excision and segmentectomy are common lung cancer operations but these procedures do carry a higher risk of the cancer coming back. According to many surgeons, if patients can tolerate a lobectomy, whereby the surgeon removes about one-third to one-half of one lung, this is the operation of choice. A lobectomy allows for the surgeon to have a greater surgical margin around the tumor. In general, removing more normal tissue around the tumor decreases the risk of the tumor coming back in this local area. At times the tumor is in the central portion of the lung or involves the major blood supply of the lung necessitating that the entire lung be removed. This procedure is called a pneumonectomy. This operation should only be performed when necessary and following a rigorous preoperative evaluation to determine if a patient's lung and heart function will tolerate the extensive operation.

Both thoracoscopy and thoracotomy are surgical approaches commonly used to provide the surgeon access to the entire chest cavity. Both operations necessitate that patients are completely asleep under general anesthesia. Thoracoscopy (or video-assisted thoracic surgery, VATS) requires the surgeon to make 2–4 small incisions over the ribcage. A small camera is placed through one of these incisions so that the surgeon can see the lung and other structures within the chest. Small instruments are inserted through the other incisions and the surgeon performs the surgical procedure with these instruments. In contrast, a thoracotomy involves a single, larger incision along the ribcage that is big enough for the surgeon to both see and place a hand within the chest. Many surgical procedures for lung cancer can be performed in a similar fashion with either approach. While thoracoscopy can lead to less pain following surgery and a shorter stay in the hospital, many patient-related and cancer-related factors help determine which approach is better for a particular patient. Your surgeon will likely discuss these options with you.

Both thoracoscopy and thoracotomy allow a thoracic surgeon the ability to remove the lung tumor and evaluate the lymph nodes within the chest. All of the types of procedures described previously (wedge excision, segmentectomy, and lobectomy) can be performed using either thoracoscopy or thoracotomy.

Both procedures require that an anesthesiologist place patients on a breathing machine or ventilator. These support devices are usually removed in the operating room but some patients will require support for longer periods of time. In addition, one chest tube also will be placed during the operation. The chest tube serves as a drain in the space between the outside of the lung and the rib cage. This tube is connected to a small device that collects fluid and allows air to escape. The chest tube remains in place until only a small amount of fluid is draining and the remaining lung has adequately re-inflated following surgery. Patients are typically walking the day following surgery and can expect to stay in the hospital for about 3–5 days.

Regardless of whether a wedge excision, segmentectomy, lobectomy, or pneumonectomy is performed, the surgeon will also evaluate lymph nodes in the chest and around the windpipe to assist with cancer staging. This often can be completed during the same surgical procedure.

Rarely, surgery may be necessary to help relieve the pain caused by a lung tumor that is otherwise too advanced for surgical removal. Advances in radiation therapy and other special treatments are often effective in reducing tumor-related pain and these modalities have reduced the need for surgery as a palliative procedure.

RECOVERY FROM SURGERY

Following surgery for lung cancer, patients typically remain in the hospital for 3–5 days. The major focus is on pain control so that patients are comfortable enough to cough, take deep breaths, and begin walking the day after surgery. All patients require oxygen initially, but most do not need oxygen after a few days. Prior to discharge from the hospital, patients should have necessary follow-up appointments with the surgeon and or medical/radiation oncologists.

Once discharged home or to a rehabilitation center, patients should have relatively few restrictions. Patients are encouraged to increase their physical activity level gradually but continually. For instance, taking a walk outside or climbing a flight of stairs are particularly good forms of exercise. Typically the main restriction for patients is to avoid lifting more than about 10–15 pounds. Generally patients are able to shower once they have been discharged from the hospital. Most patients can expect to be taking some form of pain medication for the first 1–2 weeks following surgery, but most will feel like they are back to their baseline within 10–14 days after surgery. Full recovery takes approximately 4–6 weeks. At the time of follow-up with the thoracic surgeon, if all is well, most patients will have no further restrictions and are encouraged to remain active.

SECTION 2: RADIATION THERAPY
RUSSELL HALES, MD; AND DANNY SONG, MD

Perhaps you or a loved one has been told that radiation therapy will be a part of the treatment plan. The purpose of this section is to teach the basics of radiation that every lung cancer patient should know. Your radiation oncologist will answer any specific questions you may have about the radiation.

Radiation therapy (or RT or XRT) is the use of high energy X-rays (also called photons) to treat disease. The photons are similar to those given when an X-ray or CT scan is done, but at a much higher energy. Like a flashlight beam, the photons are aimed at the tumor. The energy is high enough that most of the dose passes through the skin surface and deposits the radiation deep within the chest at the site of the tumor. This allows the skin to be spared the effects of radiation, while still giving a full dose of radiation to the tumor.

USES OF RADIATION IN LUNG CANCER

TREATING CANCER IN THE CHEST

Radiation may be given to treat lung cancer at its initial site instead of surgery if the tumor is locally advanced, but inoperable. This means that the tumor has not spread to other parts of the body but cannot be removed from the lung. If a tumor rests near or invades normal parts of the body that a patient cannot live without (such as the heart), the tumor is considered inoperable. In this case, radiation treatment is given alone or in combination with chemotherapy to treat the primary tumor. The purpose of the radiation treatment is to cause the tumor cells to die. In some situations, radiation therapy may be used to shrink the tumor enough so that excision of the tumor is then possible.

Sometimes radiation is given after surgery even if the entire tumor has been removed. This approach is utilized when patients have large or advanced tumors or when the tumor involves lymph nodes of the central chest. Even with a successful surgery, previous studies have shown that some patients may have a 40% chance of tumor recurrence in the area where it was removed. This is because cancer cells may have spread to the area surrounding the primary cancer. A successful surgery can remove all visible cancer cells, but may not remove these microscopic tumor cells. In these situations, radiation will reduce the chance of the tumor growing back in the chest.

TREATING SITES OF TUMOR SPREAD

Lung cancer can spread outside of the chest and start to grow in other areas of the body. The tumor may spread through the bloodstream and has a tendency to go to the brain, bones, or adrenal glands (small glands that sit on top of the kidneys). If tumor grows in the bone, it may cause pain in and weaken the bone. In some cases, the tumor can weaken the strong outer shell of the bone called the cortex and this may lead to a bone break or fracture. If the tumor grows in the brain, it may cause headaches or symptoms specific to the part of the brain in which it grows. These symptoms may include seizures, weakness of an arm or a leg, changes in memory, or having difficulty speaking or understanding words. Tumor spread to the adrenal glands often does not cause any symptoms, but sometimes may cause pain or abnormal function of the kidneys.

If the cancer has spread to one of these areas, radiation can be helpful in reducing the irritation caused by the tumor, shrink the tumor, and/or reduce pain in the area. For brain metastases, radiation can help relieve the symptoms and brain swelling caused by the tumor. These are the primary goals of radiation delivered to areas of metastasis. Generally, the radiation dose used will not be sufficient to completely kill all of the cancer cells at these sites of disease but will be helpful to control the tumor and some of the local side effects it may cause.

PREVENTING SPREAD TO THE BRAIN

Sometimes radiation may be given to the brain as a preventive measure, even if scans show no tumor there. Radiation oncologists call this prophylactic cranial irradiation, or PCI. With some types of lung cancer, especially SCLC, half of patients will develop tumor spread to the brain within 2 years after diagnosis. This is because tumor cells are able to spread to the brain, but the blood–brain barrier prevents many chemotherapy drugs from getting into the brain to kill these cancer cells. The brain becomes what is sometimes called a "sanctuary site" for tumor cells.

Fortunately, radiation is not affected by the blood–brain barrier. Sometimes, a lung cancer patient who has a good response to initial treatment may be surprised to learn his/her doctor is recommending brain radiation even when there is no evidence of tumor in the brain. Studies have shown that in some types of lung cancer, preventative radiation to the brain can reduce the chance of eventually developing tumor spread to the brain by more than half. This results in a significantly better chance of surviving lung cancer.

WHAT TO EXPECT: RADIATION TREATMENT A—Z

TREATMENT PLANNING

Lung cancer patients receive individualized cancer care throughout the treatment process. This is especially seen in radiation treatment. The radiation beams used for treatment are not a "one size fits all" therapy, but rather are custom designed for the anatomy of each patient. The radiation oncologist will meet with the patient and give formal recommendations, including whether or not radiation should be used. The radiation oncologist will then schedule the patient for a treatment planning scan (also known as a CT simulation).

The purpose of the simulation is to obtain information so that the radiation oncologist can devise an individualized radiation plan. Radiation therapists assist in the simulation procedure—they are individuals with special training in performing simulations as well as in the delivery of radiation as prescribed by the physician. During the simulation, the therapist positions the patient in a way that will be comfortable, accurate, and reproducible for each day that the patient is treated. A mold of the body may be made to assist in patient positioning. Two or three small permanent

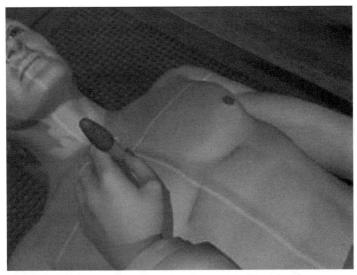

Figure 1 Marks are placed on the chest and aligned to lasers in the room to help in the precise setup of radiation treatment. Courtesy of Varian Medical Systems.

skin marks or tattoos (the size of a pen tip) will be placed on the skin to assist in precisely positioning the patient for each treatment (Figure 1). After the desired positioning is accomplished, CT images of the chest and nearby structures will be taken. These images will be used by the radiation oncologist to locate exactly where the tumor is and what important body structures need to be avoided, such as the heart and spinal cord.

The remaining process becomes more technically involved as radiation beams are arranged to meet the objectives of treating the target area, while at the same time avoiding normal structures. A team of physicists and dosimetrists (dosimetrists are team members with specialty training in radiation treatment planning) will work to design the radiation fields. The dosimetrist may place radiation beams from multiple directions (Figure 2). In addition, he or she

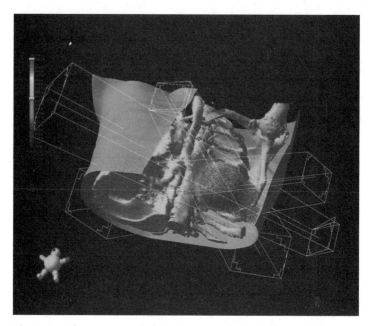

Figure 2 A lung cancer radiation treatment is designed by placing multiple beams that intersect at the tumor. Courtesy of Varian Medical Systems.

can adjust the shape of each beam to match to the shape of the target from a given direction. In some cases, the intensity of each beam can be adjusted or modulated so that a static beam can actually act as hundreds of beamlets of varying intensity. The technique to accomplish this is known as intensity modulated radiation therapy (or IMRT). The patient's radiation oncologist will determine if this form of radiation planning is right for a given tumor.

The entire process of planning, from simulation to beam arrangement, may take a few days to several weeks. The more complex the treatment plan is, the longer the amount of time necessary to plan the treatment. After quality checks are completed to ensure safe and accurate delivery of radiation, the treatment will begin.

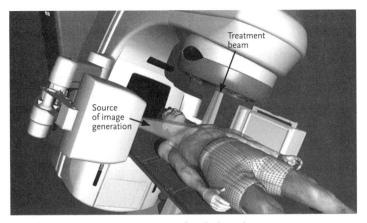

Figure 3 A patient is in position for daily radiation treatment. The treatment beam arises from the linear accelerator gantry (or arm). Images are generated to ensure correct daily positioning. Courtesy of Varian Medical Systems.

DAILY TREATMENTS

Radiation is rarely given as a single treatment. Rather, the patient with lung cancer will be given multiple small treatments of radiation over a number of days. Each daily treatment will last approximately 5–15 minutes. The actual number of radiation treatments can vary greatly depending on the plan, but upwards of 35 treatments may be given over the course of 6 weeks. The radiation oncologist will meet with the lung cancer patient weekly during treatment to answer questions, assess and treat any side effects associated with treatment, and give encouragement. If needed, most practices have a member of the radiation treatment team available daily to treat side effects that may arise during therapy.

Most radiation treatment today is delivered using a linear accelerator (Figure 3). A linear accelerator is a large machine that generates photons by accelerating electrons and directing them at a metal target. High energy X-rays are formed from this collision of the electron and the metal target in the machine. The X-rays are collected and shaped to form a beam. The beam leaves the machine through a gantry or arm that can rotate around a patient, allowing beams to be delivered from multiple different directions. In the past, radiation treatment was given by shaping the photons emitted from a radioactive substance within the treatment machine. This technique is rarely used today because there is greater safety and flexibility in generating high-energy photons with a linear accelerator.

SIDE EFFECTS: AN INTRODUCTION

Section 3 in this chapter describes in detail the possible side effects of cancer treatment, including radiation. Like all types of cancer treatment, the field of radiation oncology has experienced a tremendous degree of development in the last 10–15 years. The advances in radiation treatment have kept pace with computer technology, which allows for complex calculations and estimation of radiation dose from multiple radiation fields. The net result of this technology is an improved ability to target tumor and spare normal tissue.

In contrast to current day practice, simpler forms of radiation delivery were used to treat cancer in the past. The beams in that era were not shaped and the intensity of each beam could not be adjusted. This resulted in large treatment areas that created significant side effects and limited the effective dose of radiation that could be delivered. While it is possible that significant side effects may arise even in the modern era of radiation treatment, the probability of this toxicity is less likely today than in the past.

On a day-to-day basis, patients undergoing radiation treatment will feel no different before versus after treatment. However, depending on the specific area targeted and the organs contained in the radiation field, the treatment may gradually cause side effects over the course of treatment. Usually these side effects begin to occur after the second or third week of treatment, and then abate within a month after radiation treatment has been completed.

TARGETING TUMOR CELLS WHILE SPARING NORMAL TISSUE

Many patients ask how the radiation "knows" which cells are tumor cells and which ones are normal. Sophisticated equipment allows the radiation oncologist to direct the radiation beam at the tumor, while minimizing exposure of normal cells. However, there is normal tissue surrounding the tumor that may receive the full dose of radiation. Generally, the radiation does not kill the tumor cells directly. Instead, it damages the DNA, or genetic blueprint, of each tumor cell. When the tumor cell attempts to divide, it is unable to do so because the DNA is not readable. As a result, the tumor cell dies in the process of attempting to divide into new cancer cells.

The radiation also causes breaks in the DNA of normal cells that lie near the tumor. Do these normal cells die as well? In truth, some of these normal cells will die. However, normal cells have molecular machinery to repair damaged DNA, which may allow the healthy tissue to repair itself. This DNA repair machinery is often absent in tumor cells. Relatively small doses of radiation are given daily over many treatments (or fractions) because these small doses are more tolerable to the normal cells. That is, the dose is small enough per day that the normal cell's ability to repair itself is not exhausted. Conversely, the radiation dose, whether small or large, is likely to cause irreparable damage to tumor cells.

NEW APPROACHES AND FUTURE DIRECTIONS

While the outcomes for lung cancer have improved over the last several decades, the disease is still one where researchers are searching for therapies that will enhance survival. Clinical trials in radiation treatment provide important information to help advance the field. Your doctor may discuss these options with you.

One area of active research in radiation treatment for lung cancer is stereotactic radiation. Stereotactic radiation generally refers to administering large doses of radiation per day, which shortens the total number of radiation treatments. This approach is known as hypofractionated radiation. In order to safely give high doses per day, sophisticated radiation planning is done to deliver this high dose to the target and minimize dose to surrounding structures. Stereotactic radiation may be appropriate for small tumors that are near the outer portions of the lung (away from the central area of the chest, including the heart). The radiation oncologist will discuss with the patient whether this technique of radiation delivery is appropriate in a given context.

Some researchers are investigating the use of hyperfractionated radiation, which is the use of more than one treatment given per day, as a means of increasing the dose to the tumor while sparing normal tissue. Additionally, methods are being developed to adjust for the movement of the tumor during treatment due to breathing, such as a breath hold technique or respiratory gating. These areas of research may not only hold the potential for better outcomes in lung cancer, but may also reduce the probability of side effects from the radiation treatment.

Section 3: Chemotherapy, Treatment, and Supportive and Palliative Care
Rosalyn Juergens, MD

CHEMOTHERAPY

Chemotherapy, unlike surgery and radiation, is a systemic treatment. Surgery only affects the cancer cells that the surgeon removes, and radiation therapy only affects the cancer cells that are in the area that is being radiated. Chemotherapy reaches the bloodstream and goes where blood flow goes and, therefore, circulates through the whole system, attacking cancer cells in multiple locations. It is the most effective approach when the cancer is found in more than one location, such as in the original lung tumor and lymph nodes, or has spread into distant locations, such as the other lung, the liver, or the bones.

Chemotherapy can be given both by mouth and through the vein. The goal of the chemotherapy is to kill the cancer cells but it alone does not often offer a cure for patients with lung cancer. Chemotherapy has been shown to both prolong survival from the lung cancer as well as improve symptoms from the cancer. Chemotherapy also can be given in combination with radiation. The combination serves two purposes: the chemotherapy goes out into the bloodstream in an effort to kill off any cancer cells that may have entered into the blood stream, and it also helps the radiation do a better job of killing the cancer cells. Oncologists call this radiation sensitization.

The way chemotherapy is given varies depending on the drug used. Chemotherapy is given in rounds also known as cycles. Each cycle of chemotherapy is generally 3 or 4 weeks. Some chemotherapy combinations are given on only the first day of each cycle while others are weekly. Topoisomerase inhibitors require the most frequent treatments with either 3 or 5 straight days of chemotherapy administration.

CHEMOTHERAPY PROCESSES AND EFFECTS

Standard chemotherapy drugs generally affect cells in the body that are making copies of themselves. The hope is that the chemotherapy affects the cancer cells that are actively making copies. The classic side effects of chemotherapy are due to the fact that normal cells also make copies of themselves and they are also affected by the treatment. Some of the most common side effects from chemotherapy include hair loss because hair cells are always dividing; effects on the gastrointestinal tract including mouth sores, nausea and vomiting, and diarrhea; and lowering of the blood counts (blood is constantly being replaced).

Three main types of cells are found in the blood: red blood cells, white blood cells, and platelets. Red blood cells carry oxygen. When red blood cells are reduced, the heart needs to beat faster in order to deliver oxygen to all the tissues, especially during any physical activity. The main symptoms of a low red blood cell count are fatigue and shortness of breath. If red blood cells get too low from chemotherapy, patients can be at risk for heart attacks or strokes. Patients with low red blood cells (a condition called anemia) may require a blood transfusion.

White blood cells fight infection. Lowering the white blood cell count places patients at increased risk of infection. If patients get an infection while the blood counts are low, the infection can be life threatening. Patients need to take precautions, such as frequent hand washing and avoiding other people who are known to be sick, to reduce their risk of getting an infection. If patients who are on chemotherapy and may potentially have low blood counts develop a fever, they should be evaluated urgently to assess for signs or symptoms of infection and to be started on broad-spectrum antibiotics. Generally these patients are admitted to the hospital for monitoring and intravenous antibiotics.

Platelets are the blood cells that help blood to clot. When platelets are low, patients are at increased risk of bleeding. Patients should notify the doctor right away if they show signs of bleeding such as nosebleeds, significant bruising, or blood in the stool or urine. Each of these could represent critically low platelet counts and the patient may require a platelet transfusion.

TYPES OF CHEMOTHERAPY

Several types of chemotherapy have been developed. Chemotherapy is not one size fits all. Following you will find descriptions of the most commonly used chemotherapies for lung cancer. The choice of which chemotherapy drugs are right for you will be made after a discussion between you and your oncologist. Flexibility is available in the choice of the initial chemotherapy treatment, especially in patients who have incurable lung cancer. Informing your doctor about your other medical problems, as well as your goals of care, will be important in making the best choice.

Platinums

One of the first chemotherapy treatments available for lung cancer was a drug called Platinol-AQ (cisplatin). Platinol-AQ is still one of the most effective chemotherapies available, but it has many side effects. Hair generally falls out. Nausea and vomiting were a huge problem until modern anti-vomiting treatments became available. Kidneys can become damaged, so doctors now give lots of intravenous fluids and recommend that patients drink plenty of liquids at home. At high doses, patients can get ringing in the ears as well as high-frequency hearing loss. Platinol-AQ affects the bone marrow so patients have lowering of the blood counts (white blood cells, red blood cells, and platelets), which can lead to infection, fatigue, and bleeding. Nerves also can be damaged, causing numbness and tingling in the hands and feet. Because of the side effects, oncologists would have stopped using Platinol-AQ long ago, but it remains one of the most powerful drugs used to treat all types of lung cancer.

Paraplatin (carboplatin) is another platinum chemotherapy that was developed to be an easier to tolerate version of Platinol-AQ. Paraplatin is easier to administer to patients and the treatment takes less time (30 minutes in comparison to 4–6 hours). The side effects are also milder. Hair often does not fall out, the vomiting is much easier to treat, kidneys are less likely to be damaged, and nerves are less likely to be affected. However, paraplatin is harder on the blood counts, so patients are at a higher risk of infection and bleeding. For those patients, a discussion needs to take place comparing the risks and benefits of treatment. For many patients the ease of administration together with fewer side effects outweighs the small reduction in potency against the cancer.

Platinum chemotherapy is useful in both NSCLC and SCLC. Platinums tend to be the first chemotherapy chosen when selecting a two-drug chemotherapy combination. The second chemotherapy agent chosen tends to come from one of the following groups.

Taxanes

Currently two chemotherapy drugs in the taxane family are Food and Drug Administration- (FDA) approved for use in NSCLC. The first taxane approved was Taxol (paclitaxel). Taxol is actually a natural product, and is isolated from the Pacific Yew tree. The other taxane chemotherapy is Taxotere (docetaxel), a relative of Taxol. Because these drugs are not water soluble, the chemotherapy is dissolved in a solvent so the taxanes can be given intravenously. One of the most important side effects of taxane therapy is a risk of allergic reaction. Most patients are allergic to the solvent rather than the chemotherapy itself, so in order to try to prevent the allergic reaction associated with this class of drugs, steroids are given. Use of steroids can be very difficult in diabetic or pre-diabetic patients. Other common side effects of taxane therapy are hair loss, vomiting, decrease in blood counts, as well as significant nerve injury. Both Taxol and Taxotere can be safely combined with the platinum chemotherapies. Taxanes and platinums are given on the first day of each three-week cycle. Taxotere is one of three chemotherapies approved for use in patients who have been treated with previous chemotherapy and whose cancer has re-grown. One of the additional benefits of the taxanes is that they can be used in combination with Platinol-AQ and radiation for treatment of certain stages of lung cancer.

Vinca Alkaloids

Several chemotherapies belong to the class of drugs known as the vinca alkaloids. The name vinca alkaloids came from the fact that all the drugs in this class were derived from plants from the vinca family, which many patients are familiar with as a common flower. The most common vinca alkaloid used in NSCLC is Navelbine (vinorelbine).

The main side effects of Navelbine include hair loss, nausea and vomiting, constipation, numbness and tingling of the nerves in the hands and feet, as well as lowering of the blood counts. Another side effect of Navelbine is irritation of small veins. In order to safely administer Navelbine, a larger IV should be put in place that accesses one of the large veins (see the section in Chapter 3 on interventional radiology). Navelbine is used more in Europe and Canada than in the United States, but it is gaining popularity in combination with Platinol-AQ for use in patients after they have had surgery for their early stage lung cancer. Several large trials have shown Navelbine and Platinol-AQ is a powerful chemotherapy combination in this setting. Navelbine is given on a weekly basis in combination with platinum-based chemotherapy.

Anti-Metabolites

Several chemotherapy agents fall into the class known as anti-metabolites. Two of these drugs are commonly used in NSCLC. The first drug discovered is an agent called Gemzar (gemcitabine). The main side effects of Gemzar are reactions to the infusion including low-grade fever or achiness, and significant lowering of the blood counts. Gemzar generally produces vomiting and little hair loss. Gemzar is commonly given in combination with either of the platinums. Because of the relatively mild side effect profile, Gemzar is often chosen for use in the elderly, as well as in combination with Paraplatin for patients who are reluctant to take chemotherapy for fear of hair loss. One of the down sides of Gemzar is that the schedule requires patients to come in for treatment 2 out of every 3 weeks in the cycle.

The other commonly used anti-metabolite is Alimta (pemetrexed). Alimta is the newest standard chemotherapy available for lung cancer. The side effects of Alimta include numbness and tingling in the hands and feet, lowering of the blood counts, as well as fatigue. Hair loss is less common. Some of the side effects of Alimta can be prevented by pre-treatment of patients with injections of vitamin B12 and folic acid. Alimta was initially approved for use in patients who have been treated with chemotherapy previously and the cancer has regrown. Recently Alimta has been successfully combined with platinum chemotherapy for use in the initial treatment of lung cancer. Alimta is given on the first day of each three-week cycle.

Topoisomerase Inhibitors

Several chemotherapy drugs belong to the class known as topoisomerase inhibitors. Three are commonly used in treatment of either SCLC or NSCLC. Etopophos (etoposide) was the first topoisomerase inhibitor used in lung cancer. Etopophos in combination with platinum chemotherapy is the first choice for treatment of SCLC. Etopophos along with Platinol-AQ is the most common chemotherapy combination used with radiation for any type of lung cancer. The main side effects of Etopophos are lowering of the blood counts; gastrointestinal effects such as vomiting, constipation or diarrhea; and low blood pressure associated with dizziness.

A second topoisomerase inhibitor is Hycamtin (topotecan). Hycamtin is commonly used for patients with SCLC that has recurred after initial treatment. The main side effects of Hycamtin are significant lowering of the blood counts as well as vomiting and diarrhea. Both Etopophos and Hycamtin are available in oral and intravenous varieties.

The most recent topoisomerase inhibitor developed is Camptozar (irinotecan). Camptozar can be used in combination with platinum chemotherapy to treat both NSCLC and SCLC. Camptozar also can be used in patients with SCLC after the cancer has regrown following treatment with Etopophos and platinum chemotherapy. The main side effects of Camptozar are significant lowering of the blood counts as well as severe diarrhea.

NSCLC TREATMENT BY STAGE

Stage I

Treatment for stage I NSCLC is focused on removal of the tumor, preferably by surgery. Radiation or radiofrequency ablation (see later section) also can be used in patients for whom surgery is not an option. For most patients, additional therapy beyond surgery is not needed, but oncologists may discuss chemotherapy after surgery in patients with high-risk tumors. Further research is being done to help select which patients with stage I lung cancer should receive chemotherapy after surgery.

Stage II

Ideally, stage II NSCLC is treated with surgery followed by chemotherapy. Approximately half of all stage II NSCLC patients treated with surgery alone will have their tumors return. Chemotherapy given after surgery can reduce that risk.

Stage III

Treatment of stage III NSCLC is more complicated. Stage IIIA NSCLC can be approached in multiple ways. The most important part is that the treatment plan is arranged in a multidisciplinary group, including medical, radiation, and surgical oncology. Generally, the defining factor is whether or not the surgeon feels that the cancer can safely be removed with surgery and, if so, what type of surgery will be required. For stage IIIA NSCLC, chemotherapy, radiation, and surgery are often all used. For stage IIIA NSCLC patients with cancers that cannot be safely removed, or for patients with stage IIIB NSCLC, combined chemotherapy and radiation are the mainstay of therapy.

Stage IV

Stage IV NSCLC, by definition, is lung cancer that has spread to distant parts of the body. The best approach for these patients is chemotherapy. Surgery is generally not recommended. Radiation is used to treat symptoms such as painful spread to the bones, tumors in the brain, or narrowed airways in the lungs. Chemotherapy for a patient with NSCLC who has not already received chemotherapy is generally given as a pair of drugs. Often one drug comes from the platinum class of chemotherapies. Research has shown that one standard chemotherapy alone in the first line offers less benefit than two chemotherapies put together. Three standard chemotherapies put together often give patients more side effects and do not offer better response or survival. In addition, targeted therapies (see pages 49–50) may be added to the standard chemotherapy. Once a patient has cancer that grows after receiving the first type of treatment, doctors often use one chemotherapy drug or targeted treatment at a time.

SCLC TREATMENT BY STAGE

Limited Stage SCLC

Limited stage SCLC is small cell lung cancer that is confined to one lung and the lymph nodes in the lung. The way this was initially defined was SCLC that could be safely treated all in one radiation field. With improvements in radiation technology, the number of patients who fall into this category has increased. The new technology has allowed radiation oncologists to more easily focus the radiation beams on areas of cancer while sparing more normal lung. The key to treating and curing limited stage SCLC is administering both chemotherapy and radiation therapy at the same time. Often chemotherapy will begin first since chemotherapy can normally be arranged within 24 hours. Radiation should start by the second cycle of therapy. Generally 4 cycles of chemotherapy are given along with radiation. The optimal maximum dose and schedule of radiation for SCLC is up for debate. Research has shown that twice daily radiation may offer better survival than once daily radiation, but patients and treatment centers often have difficulty making arrangements for this type of intensive treatment. When once daily radiation is given, higher doses of radiation are used. Patients are often treated with radiation to the brain and chest after completing chemotherapy. Spread to the brain is very common in SCLC so in order to kill any microscopic cancer cells that may have spread to the brain, preventive radiation is used.

Extensive Stage SCLC

Extensive stage SCLC is defined as small cell lung cancer that cannot be treated safely in one radiation field. The standard for treatment of extensive stage SCLC is combined chemotherapy. Generally, the first treatment is a combination of Etopophos and either Platinol-AQ or Paraplatin. Because of the nature of extensive stage disease, the cancer usually recurs, and treatment in a clinical trial is often recommended. However, chemotherapy is effective for palliation and can decrease symptoms and extend the quality of a patient's life.

TARGETED THERAPIES

Standard chemotherapy generally relies upon the fact that cancer cells are frequently making copies of themselves, but many normal cells are also making copies of themselves on a daily basis. The effects of chemotherapy on those normal cells lead to many of the typical side effects of standard chemotherapy such as hair loss, nausea, diarrhea, and low blood counts. Cancer research has been moving forward to try to develop cancer treatments that are more specific or "targeted" at the cancer cells themselves, sparing more of the normal healthy cells.

The first targeted treatment that became available for NSCLC was Iressa (gefitinib). Iressa belongs to a class of drugs called epidermal growth factor receptor (EGFR) inhibitors. The epidermal growth factor pathway is associated with the growth, survival, and spread of lung cancer. Blocking this pathway in some patients slows the growth of the cancer. In patients with specific abnormalities in the EGFR, EGFR inhibitors can lead to impressive response to the therapy. A newer, more potent agent, Tarceva (erlotinib), has replaced Iressa as the main EGFR inhibitor prescribed in North America after a clinical trial showed improved survival for patients with lung cancer that had grown despite previous treatment with platinum-based chemotherapy. Further research is being done on how best to select patients for treatment with EGFR inhibitors as well as the optimal timing for their use. Both Iressa and Tarceva are treatments that are available in pill form. A third drug, Erbitux (cetuximab), is an intravenous drug that targets this same pathway. Erbitux is currently approved for use in colon cancer and head and neck cancer, and is being studied for use with chemotherapy in lung cancer.

The next targeted therapy that was approved for lung cancer attacks the ability of the tumor(s) to develop their own blood vessels. Avastin (bevacizumab) is an intravenous drug that absorbs the signal that cancer cells send out to try to make new blood vessels. Avastin is approved for use in combination with platinum-based chemotherapy as part of the initial therapy for non-squamous NSCLC that has spread through the bloodstream to other sites. The addition of Avastin to chemotherapy has significantly improved the ability of treatment to shrink the cancer cells as well as improved survival for patients with advanced lung cancer. Avastin does have side effects including risk of serious bleeding, as well as thickening of the blood, which could lead to serious blood clots, heart attacks, and strokes. High blood pressure is also a common side effect of this therapy. For many patients, the benefits outweigh the risks of therapy.

Numerous other targeted therapies for lung cancer are currently under investigation. Clinical trials are being conducted throughout the world trying to discover therapies that will improve the survival of lung cancer patients as well as improve their quality of life while on the therapy.

INTERVENTIONAL PULMONARY AND RADIOLOGY
PROCEDURES

New technologies are also being used in the fight against
lung cancer. Under certain circumstances, procedures may
be recommended to add to your cancer care. Certain techniques may improve the symptoms of your cancer, aid in the
delivery of your chemotherapy, or attack the cancer itself.

Procedures For Improving Symptoms From The Cancer

• *Thoracentesis and Pleural Catheter Placement.* Lung
  cancer patients may have involvement of the lining
  around the lung by cancer cells. When the lining of
  the lung is irritated by cancer cells, the response of the
  body is to make fluid. This fluid accumulates in the
  space between the lung and the chest wall called the
  pleural space. This condition is called a pleural
  effusion. Small amounts of this fluid do not cause
  symptoms, but when a large amount of fluid is present, significant breathing troubles can be present. The
  main treatment to relieve the shortness of breath from
  fluid around the lung is to drain the fluid using a
  needle. This procedure is called a thoracentesis and is
  generally a safe procedure that can be done in the
  clinic at the bedside or under ultrasound guidance.
  The risks of a thoracentesis are infection, bleeding,
  and pneumothorax (a collapse of a lung or portion
  of the lung). When patients have fluid that reaccu-
  mulates quickly after a thoracentesis, consideration
  should be given for a more permanent solution. One
  option is placing a piece of tubing into the pleural
  space to allow frequent drainage. The most common
  catheter used for this purpose is a Pleurx catheter.
  Placement of a Pleurx catheter allows patients to drain

fluid at home, on a daily basis if needed, without the risks of needle insertion from a thoracentesis. With time, these catheters can cause the lining around the lung to become stuck to the chest wall, which decreases the amount of fluid created. Eventually this may allow the catheter to be removed.

Alternatively, a surgeon can remove the fluid in the operating room and place talc or other materials in the space between the lung and the ribcage. This procedure is called pleurodesis. The goal of the procedure is to cause an irritation within the outer lining of the lung and the ribcage so that the two layers stick together and prevent fluid from building up. While this procedure involves an operation and requires a hospital stay, it does avoid the need for a long-term catheter and home fluid drainage.

- *Vascular Stenting*. Major blood vessels that enter and exit the heart and lungs are located in the center of the chest. Sometimes lung cancers or lymph nodes, which are involved with lung cancer, are located in the center of the chest. When these tumors become large enough, they can compress the blood vessels. The most commonly affected blood vessel is called the superior vena cava (SVC). When the SVC is blocked, the face and arms can become swollen due to back up of the blood that should be draining into the heart. SVC blockage may be a life-threatening emergency. In order to attempt to open this blood vessel, a balloon is inflated to open up the narrowed area and a small wire mesh tube called a stent is permanently placed in the newly opened artery or vein to help it remain open. Stenting is often performed to allow your doctor to begin chemotherapy and/or radiation to try to shrink the lung cancer.

- *Bronchial and Tracheal Stenting.* When you breathe in air, the air travels through a large breathing tube, called the trachea, which then splits off to bring air to the right and left lungs through tubes called the bronchi. Sometimes cancers grow along the trachea or bronchi and block these tubes. When a tube is blocked, air has greater difficulty getting past the blockage, which can lead to more difficulty breathing or pneumonia in the area of the lung behind the blockage. In order to allow air to enter into that area of the lung, a wire mesh stent can be placed to open up that airway. Stents are placed by pulmonologists, surgeons, or other trained specialists during a procedure called a bronchoscopy. To perform a bronchoscopy, the doctor takes a tube with a camera and a light on the end of it and looks into the airway. Through that tube, a stent can be placed. Stents come with risks such as bleeding, creation of holes in the airway, and infection, so they are normally only used for major, life-threatening blockages.

- *Radiofrequency Ablation.* Radiofrequency ablation (RFA) is a minimally invasive treatment for cancer. In radiofrequency ablation, imaging techniques such as ultrasound, CT scans, or MRIs are used to help guide a needle electrode into a cancerous tumor. High-frequency electrical currents are then passed through the electrode, creating heat that destroys the abnormal cells. RFA is generally only used in those patients who are not candidates for surgical removal of their lung cancer. The best results are in patients who have small tumors and do not have lymph node involvement from the cancer. The main risk of the procedure is collapse of the lung when the needle is placed into the tumor. Only certain tumors are treatable with RFA. Tumors too close to the heart or major blood vessels cannot be safely treated due to risk to these important structures.

53

Procedures To Help Administer Treatment:
Vascular Catheter Placement

Most chemotherapy is given through the veins. Often patients are in the clinic at least on a weekly basis for laboratory tests or treatments. Frequent blood draws and IV placements can be difficult on patients. Certain chemotherapies also can be hard or even dangerous to give through standard IVs. Before beginning chemotherapy, your doctor may recommend that you have a more permanent IV placed to allow for easy access into your blood stream for blood testing or administration of chemotherapy or intravenous fluids. Several types of these catheters are available.

Mediports or ports are catheters that are placed under the skin. Ports are inserted under the skin through a small incision and are connected to a piece of tubing that is inserted into a large blood vessel either in the neck or under the collarbone. Ports are convenient because, when they are not in use, nothing is left outside the body. Ports can last many years. In order to gain entry to the blood stream through a port, a needle is inserted through the skin into the hub of the port. The needle is then connected to tubing through which fluids or chemotherapy are given. The down side is that they are more challenging to remove if a problem develops with the port, such as malfunction, infection, or a blood clot.

Hickman and Groshong catheters are intravenous catheters that tunnel underneath a portion of the skin and into the large blood vessel in the neck or under the collarbone. Unlike a port, these catheters have tubing that comes out of the skin. The portion of the catheter that is outside the body dangles on the chest. A needle is not required to gain access to the bloodstream through these catheters. These catheters are easy to remove in an emergency and are used most frequently in blood cancers but can be used for lung cancer patients as well.

Peripherally inserted central catheters (PICC) are catheters placed into the large blood vessel in the arm rather than the large blood vessels in the neck or chest. PICC lines also have a portion of the line that is outside of the body and normally is kept covered on the upper part of the arm. The benefit of PICC lines is that they avoid the risk of allowing air to enter into the lung space during insertion, which can cause collapse of the lung called a pneumothorax. Because the lung lies underneath the blood vessel under the collarbone as well as at the bottom of the neck, a small risk of lung collapse exists when inserting either ports or either of the tunneled catheters. PICC lines may be the best catheter in patients with severe emphysema because collapse of the lung could have severe side effects. PICC lines are also easy to remove.

CLINICAL TRIALS

Clinical trials are studies in which people volunteer to test new drugs or procedures. Doctors use clinical trials to learn whether a new treatment is safe and effective in humans. These studies are necessary for developing new treatments for serious diseases such as lung cancer. Clinical trial participants also help future patients who are diagnosed with lung cancer by helping to improve how we treat lung cancer.

Clinical Trial Phases

A new drug or procedure needs to undergo extensive testing before being approved by the Food and Drug Administration (FDA) for general use. New treatments proceed through each of three phases of clinical trials before a decision is made by the FDA for approval. For the purposes of this discussion, we will focus on the development of new chemotherapy drugs, but a similar process is used to develop new uses for radiation or interventional techniques.

Patients who participate in clinical trials are among the first to receive new treatments before they are widely available. However, there is no guarantee that the new treatment will be safe, effective, or better than a standard treatment. Patients decide to participate in clinical trials for many reasons. Your doctors may discuss with you opportunities to participate in a clinical trial at any given time during your treatment. Be open-minded. For some patients, a clinical trial is the best treatment option available. Because standard treatments are not perfect, patients are often willing to face the added uncertainty of a clinical trial in the hope of a better result. Other patients volunteer for clinical trials because they know that this is the only way to make progress in treating lung cancer. Even if they do not benefit directly from the clinical trial, their participation may benefit future people with lung cancer.

> *Phase I* clinical trial goals are for a new drug are
> to establish what a safe dose of the drug is and the
> schedule of the drug, or how often the drug should
> be given. Another goal of a phase I study is to assess
> what side effects the drug produces in humans.
> Pre-clinical testing, or testing in animals, can help
> doctors to estimate a safe starting dose and schedule
> for these trials. Participation in a phase I clinical trial
> often requires frequent blood tests or even biopsies
> of the cancer or other tissues such as skin. These tests
> help the doctors conducting the trial to make deci-
> sions about how to proceed during the trial. Phase I
> clinical trials change as new information is gathered
> from patients who are enrolled. The first patients

enrolled in a phase I trial are likely to get a much lower dose of the new drug than those who are enrolled in later phases of the trial. Often phase I trials are open to patients with different types of cancer. Patients with different types of cancer can be enrolled because phase I studies are not looking at tumor response or patient survival as a main goal. Because response is not the primary goal, the type of tumor the patient has is less important. In general, the reported response rate (defined as shrinkage of the tumor by at least 50%) in phase I clinical trials conducted through the National Cancer Institute in the last 10 years is approximately 5%.

Phase I clinical trials are not only focused on new drugs that are coming straight out of the research laboratory. Phase I clinical trials are also done when doctors are trying to combine two drugs, even if both of those drugs are already FDA approved. Many phase I clinical trials look at what the correct dose and schedule is for these new combinations, as well as if the new combination has a safe side effect profile. This type of phase I clinical trial is very appealing to patients, especially when one of the drugs in the clinical trial is a drug that they would already be receiving as part of standard of care for their lung cancer. For some patients, their first chemotherapy treatment may be part of a phase I clinical trial if the study is assessing standard treatment plus a new drug.

Phase II clinical trials are designed to assess what the impact is of a new drug or drug combination on a particular tumor type. For these trials, each patient on the study generally receives the same dose of chemotherapy. The outcome of the trial is generally measured as either the percentage of patients whose tumor shrinks from the treatment (response rate) or the amount of time before the cancer grows more than 20% (time to progression). A phase II clinical trial is considered successful if there is an increase in either response or time to progression as compared to what we would normally expect from other available drugs given in that setting. The amount of increase the physicians consider as important enough to take to the next step changes depending on the stage of the patients in the trial, as well as the number of previous treatments the patients have received.

Phase III clinical trials are the final stage of testing for a new drug. In a phase III clinical trial, a new treatment is compared directly to another, older treatment that is considered the standard of care. In order to do this comparison, patients are enrolled into one of at least 2 groups. Some trials have more than 2 groups if there are several treatments considered standard or if more than one experimental treatment is being compared to the standard treatment. In order to determine which of the treatments each patient will get, a process called randomization is used. Randomization allows each patient at the time of study entry to have a random chance of being entered on each of the treatment arms (like flipping a coin). The goal of a phase III clinical trial is to compare the survival between two treatments. Survival in phase III clinical trials is our best evidence comparing available therapies. Other outcomes such as response or time to progression are just shorter term substitutes for what we really want to know: who lives longer?

Patients who are interested in clinical trials should mention this to their doctors each time they are discussing changes in treatment. The participation of patients in clinical trials brings us closer each day to a cure for lung cancer. Research in lung cancer is not limited to just clinical trials with new drugs, radiation techniques, or surgeries. Many types of research exist. Filling out surveys on quality of life or donating blood or tumor cells for use in investigating new treatments in the laboratory are just some ways patients can also provide critical assistance in our fight against lung cancer.

SUPPORTIVE CARE

ALTERNATIVE/COMPLEMENTARY MEDICINE

Complementary and alternative medicine (CAM), as defined by the NIH's National Center for Complementary and Alternative Medicine (NCCAM), is a group of diverse medical and healthcare practices and products that are not presently considered to be part of conventional medicine. Conventional medicine is generally accepted as medicine that is practiced by holders of MD (medical doctor) or DO (doctor of osteopathy) degrees and by their allied health professionals, such as physical therapists, psychologists, and registered nurses. Some healthcare providers practice both CAM and conventional medicine. Complementary medicine can be used together with conventional medicine, while alternative medicine is used in place of conventional medicine. Nearly half of all cancer patients report use of some form of CAM as part of their approach to cancer treatment.

Acupuncture

Acupuncture is a technique of inserting fine needles into specific points on the body with the aim of relieving pain or for other therapeutic purposes. Acupuncture is being studied for treatment of cancer-related pain, as well as chemotherapy-associated nausea and vomiting. Many cancer centers offer access to reputable practitioners of acupuncture. Patients who are undergoing chemotherapy need to consult their doctor before starting acupuncture to ensure that they are not at increased risk of bleeding due to low platelets or blood thinners.

Dietary, Herbal, and Vitamin Supplements

The most common form of CAM is the usage of dietary, herbal, and vitamin supplements. If you are taking any of these supplements, make a complete list of what you are taking and the amount. Many supplements can interact in harmful ways with other medicines, so talk with your doctor and pharmacist about your supplements. Report any changes in your supplement use to your healthcare team. Many cancer centers have access to nutritionists who can be useful guides in managing your nutritional needs during and after cancer treatment. In general, eating a well balanced diet is a good start for most cancer patients.

Meditation and Spiritual Support

Spirituality has many forms and can be practiced in many ways. Prayer may be silent or spoken out loud, alone, or in groups. Spirituality also can be practiced without a formal religion. Some people express their spirituality by spending time with nature, doing creative work, or by serving others. Meditation also involves spirituality. Many medical institutions and practitioners include spirituality and prayer as important components of healing.

PALLIATIVE CARE

Palliative care is defined as care whose goal is not to cure cancer, but is aimed at relieving suffering and improving the quality of life in patients. In many respects, chemotherapy and radiation are given as palliative care. Radiation is often given to patients not in an effort to cure their cancers, but rather to address a particular problem. For example, when cancer spreads to the bones, the tumors in the bones can be painful and a few doses of radiation to the site of the painful bone can alleviate severe pain.

Bones that have cancer in them are weaker than healthy bones. Another treatment that can improve quality of life is bisphosphonate therapy. Bisphosphonates were initially designed to treat osteoporosis but the most powerful drugs in the bisphosphonate family are also effective for removing calcium from the bloodstream and helping strengthen bones by slowing bone breakdown. Use of these drugs reduces the risk of fracture from bone metastases.

For many cancer patients, breathing difficulties can lead to significant symptoms. Doctors should assess lung cancer patients for the need for oxygen. Low oxygen levels may not be obvious when tested at rest. Oxygen levels should be tested both while the patient is resting as well as when the patient is moving around. Oxygen can be obtained for use in the home and for use while away from the home (portable oxygen).

Pain is the symptom that many cancer patients fear most. Pain management is a very important part of your cancer care. Pain should be approached from multiple angles. The two initial goals should be finding the source of pain and treating the pain. These two goals need to be approached at the same time. Finding the source of the pain generally requires different types of X-rays such as CT scans, MRIs, and bone scans.

Management of the pain generally involves prescription pain medication. For non-cancer patients, standard pain medications such as Tylenol (acetaminophen) and Advil (ibuprofen) generally are good enough to treat most aches and pains. For cancer patients on chemotherapy, Tylenol and Advil may mask a fever that is an early sign of an infection. Non-steroidal anti-inflammatory drugs (NSAIDs), such as Advil, also come with other side effects such as reducing the ability of blood to clot and affecting kidney function that could be harmful to cancer patients who are receiving chemotherapy. Both Tylenol and Advil have limits in the amount of medication that can be taken safely daily, which makes them less than optimal primary pain therapy choices. Often one of the first drugs utilized to treat cancer pain comes from the class of drugs called opiates. Morphine and other opiates such as oxycodone are used commonly in cancer patients. Initially most doctors start with short-acting pain medication (medication that has effects that last 4–6 hours) in order to estimate the amount of pain medication required to control the pain of the patient. If patients are requiring pain medication on a frequent basis, long-acting pain medications are available that provide a more continuous dosing of pain medication.

Opiate pain medications are not the only options. Other pain medications called adjuncts can be added to opiates to gain additional benefits. Steroids help patients with pain from bone metastases. Tricyclic antidepressants and certain antiseizure medications such as Neurontin (gabapentin) or Lyrica (pregabalin) are useful in helping address painful burning, numbness, or tingling from nerve pain, or neuropathy. Many cancer centers have pain specialists to address cancer pain. Some of these specialists are anesthesiologists who may be able to offer nerve blocks that provide a local approach to certain types of pain.

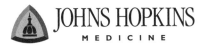

CHAPTER 4

BE PREPARED—THE SIDE EFFECTS OF TREATMENT

HONGBIN CHEN, MD, PHD; JUSTIN F. KLAMERUS, MD; AND DAVID S. ETTINGER, MD, FACP, FCCP

Despite the potential benefits, cancer treatment can also cause side effects. Just like any other medical treatment, therapies for lung cancer, including surgery, radiation therapy, chemotherapy, and targeted therapy, may bring undesirable side effects. This is because these treatments not only kill tumor cells but also affect normal cells in the body. Cells that divide rapidly (such as hair follicles, blood cells, mucosal cells lining the digestive tract, and skin cells) are commonly damaged by cancer treatment. The development of side effects mainly depends on the type, intensity, and duration of the treatment. In addition, age, general health, physical function, other medical conditions, and the severity of lung cancer are often important factors to predict side effects. For instance, studies have shown that if a lung cancer patient is confined to bed rest for most of the day due to poor health, he or she probably would not benefit from aggressive cancer treatment because the side effects of such treatment may become intolerable and may even cause death.

Concerns about potential side effects can influence the choice of the most appropriate cancer treatment for you. For example, for a lung cancer patient with underlying kidney disease, the oncologist may choose a different but equally effective chemotherapy drug to avoid the worsening of the kidney function. Patients and their family members often worry about side effects because of things they have read or things they have heard from other patients. However, it is important to realize that not all cancer patients experience the same level of side effects, even from the same treatment. Some side effects are common to different therapies, such as fatigue in patients receiving chemotherapy or radiation therapy. And some side effects may be unique to a specific treatment, such as skin reaction from the radiation therapy.

There is no doubt that we have made a lot of progress to decrease side effects of cancer treatment. For instance, radiation oncologists are able to radiate the smallest body area to minimize the toxicity to the surrounding normal tissues. Some newer generation chemotherapy drugs are much less toxic than the older ones. One area of great advancement in cancer treatment in the past two decades is supportive care. Many agents given in supportive care are not intended to cure lung cancer; instead, they help to preserve patients' overall health by treating or even preventing side effects. As our knowledge of cancer treatment increases, more and more patients are tolerating treatment with much fewer side effects. This is achieved with careful planning and effective supportive care.

Since experiencing side effects, however mild, is an inherent part of cancer treatment, the doctor must discuss both the potential benefits and side effects of a therapy with you before deciding which treatment you should receive. A surgeon will tell you the risks of an operation. A radiation oncologist will let you know about the toxicities from radiation therapy. A medical oncologist will present possible side effects from chemotherapy and novel targeted therapy. If you are eligible for a clinical study, the doctor will go over the possible risks of any treatment in the study. It is important that you are armed with as much information as you need to make your decisions. You and your family members are encouraged to take down notes or possibly record discussions during clinic visits. It is a good time for you and your loved ones to ask questions and raise concerns about treatment, and this information will help you to make an informed decision about your cancer treatment. It also helps to prepare you both physically and mentally for the road ahead. Other members of the cancer treatment team will provide related information to you as well. For instance, if you have surgery, an anesthesiologist will come to evaluate you and tell you what kind of side effects you may expect from the anesthesia procedure. At many cancer treatment centers, before a patient starts chemotherapy, the chemotherapy nurse will conduct a "chemotherapy teaching session" regarding the dos and don'ts during treatment. You can find out more information about a specific cancer treatment and its side effects from other reliable sources. Some of these resources are listed in Chapter 11.

It is important for you to follow the doctor's advice about the treatment and potential side effects and to take necessary precautions prescribed whenever indicated. For example, you may be asked to take a medication the day before the chemotherapy to prevent a side effect from a particular chemotherapy drug. During the treatment, you should immediately alert your doctor or nurse to any new discomfort or symptoms you experience while on treatment. These may be caused by or related to the cancer treatment you are receiving. Timely report of possible side effects can help the doctor to determine the cause of these events and decide whether an intervention is warranted. Adequate management of side effects can maintain your quality of life during treatment and help you through these challenged times. Most side effects can be controlled or limited, but doing so requires careful attention from patients, family, friends, and care providers. It is important to remember that if the side effects become too severe in spite of multiple attempts to control them, it may be time for you and your doctor to decide whether the treatment is hurting you more than it is helping you. New decisions may need to be made. The fact that a small minority of patients may die as a result of serious toxicities from cancer treatment further highlights the importance of an open and thorough discussion between you and your doctor so that your cancer treatment plan balances the risks and benefits.

As discussed in the previous chapter, most lung cancer patients will receive a combination of treatments, typically surgery followed by chemotherapy and/or radiation therapy. Some patients will receive chemotherapy along with radiation therapy. This combination may lead to increased chances of getting treatment-related side effects and the following sections discuss possible side effects based on different treatments, as well as the management of some common side effects that you may experience.

SURGERY

If you are considered a surgical candidate, you will undergo an extensive evaluation, including cardiopulmonary (heart and lung) function tests before the operation. Even with the best planning and safer surgical techniques, side effects from surgery of lung cancer can occur during and after the operation. Patients commonly receive general anesthesia for the surgery. Insertion of a breathing tube down the throat connected to a breathing machine, or intubation, may cause injury in the airway. Significant blood loss during the surgery can drop the blood pressure and decrease oxygen supply to the vital organs, such as the heart and brain.

After the operation, patients may need ventilator support for a short period in the critical care unit and are usually sedated during this time. The longer this period (called perioperative period), the more likely it is for some patients to develop complications, such as infections or blood clots. Blood clots usually form first in the blood vessels in the arms or legs (a condition called deep venous thrombosis) and may travel to the lungs (a condition called pulmonary embolism). The risk is higher for blood clots to form in cancer patients and those remaining immobilized in bed for an extended period of time. Knowing these risks, the doctors will always try to remove the breathing tube as soon as the patient's respiratory function recovers. The nurse and respiratory therapist will then teach the patient breathing exercises to cough out sputum and expand the remaining lungs to decrease the risk of lung infection. In order to prevent blood clots, a compressive device may be placed around the legs. The device slowly inflates and deflates, massaging the legs to prevent clot formation. In addition, an injection of a blood thinner such as heparin may be given. Early out of bed activity, whenever permitted, is encouraged. Some patients may need a short period of physical therapy and rehabilitation to help them recover after surgery.

Some pre-existing diseases can increase your risks associated with surgery. For example, diabetes can compromise the wound healing process if the blood sugars are not well controlled before, during, or after the surgery. Patients who are heavy smokers and have emphysema or COPD may require additional oxygen for a longer period.

Inevitably patients will experience pain at the surgical wound. The doctor and nurse will assess your pain level whenever necessary, usually by asking for a pain score from 0 (no pain) to 10 (most painful) on a continuous scale. This will help them to determine the best approach to control the pain. Most patients will need pain medications, either given on scheduled intervals or as needed. Stronger pain medications may be necessary to relieve post-operative pain. Some patients fear getting addicted to pain medications, but addiction is unlikely to occur when the medications are used properly for pain control under the supervision of a doctor or pharmacist. Newer generations of pain medications are more effective than the older ones and have fewer side effects. Sometimes an infusion pump is used to give a pain medication, such as morphine, continuously by the vein or under the skin. The patient can press a button to self administer extra doses of pain medication as needed—this is called the self-controlled morphine pump. Usually, it can be converted to an oral medication after the pain is better controlled. When the underlying cause of the pain is adequately addressed, most patients do not require long-term use of pain medications after the surgery. However if the pain persists despite these treatments, the patient may be referred to a pain clinic where a pain specialist can evaluate and manage the pain.

RADIATION THERAPY

Just like surgery, radiation therapy is also considered a form of local therapy to treat lung cancer. The side effects from radiation therapy often depend on where the radiation is focused on the body and how much radiation is given in total. In order to minimize side effects, radiation is typically given 5 days a week over a period of several weeks. Side effects often start by the second or third week of radiation treatment. Since radiation has cumulative effects, side effects may worsen toward the end of the treatment period. Thanks to modern radiation machines and improved techniques, the risk of damage to surrounding tissues and organs, such as healthy lung and the heart, is now markedly reduced from what may have been experienced in the past.

The skin in the radiation area may become red, dry, irritated, or tender, like a mild to moderate sunburn, and some areas may become darker later. You can wash your skin with mild soap or use a steroid or antibacterial cream or lotion if necessary. Wearing loose-fitting cotton clothes can help avoid skin irritation. If the area of skin damage becomes painful, you can take pain medication. In addition, you may experience a sore throat or develop a dry cough. Occasionally patients may have trouble swallowing as radiation to the chest harms the lining of the esophagus. A general loss of appetite during the treatment, in combination with discomfort in swallowing, may result in weight loss, so your radiation oncologist may recommend a temporary feeding tube be placed prior to starting treatment. A feeding tube is placed through the skin of the abdomen and goes directly into the stomach. This alternative path to the stomach will be used to provide necessary nutrition to maintain health during treatment; you will still be able to continue eating by mouth as you normally do.

Most patients also report feeling tired or fatigue. Taking a nap or exercising as tolerated may be an effective way to combat fatigue. Nevertheless, many patients are able to continue all or most of their routine daily activities during radiation treatment. With good supportive care, patients can usually expect to complete the radiation therapy without interruption.

For patients who receive radiation to the brain for treatment or prevention of metastatic disease from the lung cancer, mild to moderate nausea and vomiting or headache may occur. Your doctor may prescribe antivomiting medications or sometimes low-dose steroids to help with these symptoms if necessary.

Some patients are concerned that radiation therapy or chemotherapy may cause another cancer later in life. While this is possible, the risk of developing a second cancer from radiation is very low. The benefit of treating and curing cancer by radiation therapy and chemotherapy far outweighs this very small risk.

CHEMOTHERAPY

If chemotherapy is planned after surgery, usually you must wait 4–6 weeks before starting chemotherapy as it may disrupt wound healing. Likewise, you may also want to put on hold other non-urgent procedures, such as plastic surgery, until chemotherapy is completed. You should see a family doctor or a specialist if you need management of other medical conditions such as hypertension or diabetes and you should get a flu shot if it is flu season. You should also see a dentist for dental cleaning or any dental work before starting chemotherapy. It is extremely important that you tell your medical oncologist all of the prescription medications as well as over-the-counter products that you are taking. Vitamins, supplements, or herbal preparations may have significant interactions with chemotherapy. Since we know little about these drug interactions, they may have potential negative impact on chemotherapy; therefore, patients are discouraged from taking non-prescription supplements during the chemotherapy treatment.

When you hear the word chemotherapy, fears of hair loss, nausea, and vomiting may immediately come to your mind. The oncologist must understand those fears and should support you during this time. Side effects of chemotherapy primarily depend on which medication is chosen, what dosage is given, and how many cycles of treatment are received. Most side effects are predictable and typically follow an expected course. The medical team will closely monitor you for symptoms and signs of any side effects. If side effects persist and become intolerable, your doctor can adjust the dose of a chemotherapy medication or change it to another medication. Sometimes your doctor needs to postpone the next treatment in order to reduce these side effects and let you recuperate.

Common side effects from chemotherapy for treatment of lung cancer include hair loss, poor appetite, nausea, vomiting, low blood cell counts, infection, mouth sores, fatigue, skin rash, and tingling or numbness. Occasionally, serious side effects can affect liver or kidney function.

HAIR LOSS

Most chemotherapy regimens to treat lung cancer can cause hair loss, a condition called alopecia. Hair loss usually starts about a couple of weeks after the first dose of chemotherapy. You may choose to wear a wig or hat, and many insurance companies will pay for a wig if your doctor writes a prescription. Your hair will grow back after chemotherapy is completed, but sometimes your new hair may be slightly different in color or texture.

NAUSEA AND VOMITING

You may feel nauseated or may even vomit during the treatment. This often occurs during the first few days of each chemotherapy cycle, and might cause you to develop fears in anticipation of the next dose of chemotherapy. Almost all chemotherapy today incorporates 1–3 antinausea/vomiting medications, depending on the risk of vomiting associated with the chemotherapeutic regimen used. It is very important that you take these medications exactly as instructed, as some are given to treat nausea/vomiting while others may be given to prevent nausea/vomiting. Research has led to the development of newer generations of antinausea/vomiting medications that are more effective at controlling or preventing nausea/vomiting.

POOR APPETITE AND NUTRITIONAL STATUS

You may lose your appetite during the treatment and this may further decrease your energy level. You should have your weight measured on a regular basis. Controlling nausea and vomiting is important, as discussed above. Small, frequent intake of snacks or food is sometimes helpful, and you may benefit from medications that can stimulate your appetite. A consultation with a dietician can be helpful to get professional advice on how to meet your nutritional needs. If you receive chemotherapy and radiation therapy at the same time, a condition called esophagitis that causes swallowing to be very painful may occur. In addition to pain control, you may need a temporary tube inserted into your stomach or small bowel in the abdomen to provide essential nutritional support. If you are not able to take food orally or need bowel rest, your doctor may prescribe total nutritional support by infusion through your veins.

LOW BLOOD CELL COUNTS

Chemotherapy can affect all of the blood cells in the body because blood cells are rapidly dividing. Consequently, blood cell counts typically decrease within 1–2 weeks after chemotherapy treatment begins. If your red blood cell counts are low, you may tire more easily than usual or even feel short of breath. If your white blood cell counts are low (a condition called leukopenia or neutropenia), you may become more susceptible to infections. If your platelet counts are low (a condition called thrombocytopenia), you may be at risk for bruises or bleeding. During chemotherapy treatment, it is important to obtain sufficient rest and avoid physical exertion or injury. Common precautions to decrease the risk of infection, such as frequent hand washing and avoiding being around people who are sick, are important. If your platelets are low, you should also avoid certain medications such as aspirin that may prevent your platelets from working properly. In most cases, blood cell counts should return to normal levels within 1–2 weeks. Your doctor will monitor your blood counts to ensure that it is safe to start the next cycle of treatment. Occasionally, if the counts are too low or they do not return to normal as expected, your doctor may order a blood transfusion or an injection of a medication, called a growth factor, that can help your body make new blood cells.

INFECTION

As mentioned previously, your risk of infection increases when white blood cell counts are low. As a result, your body's immune system may be compromised. Patients who have other major medical conditions, such as poorly controlled diabetes, or who have a long-term infusion catheter in the body are also considered at high risk. It is important that you have a thermometer to measure your temperature whenever you feel warm or experience chills. If your white blood cell counts drop significantly after chemotherapy is started, your doctor may start antibiotics to prevent an infection.

Symptoms or signs of a potential infection include fever (temperature higher than 100.8°F); new cough or trouble breathing; headache; sinus pain; stomachache; diarrhea; pain or burning with urination; or redness, swelling, warmth, or pain in any body part. If you are experiencing these symptoms, you should call a doctor or nurse immediately. Frequently, the doctor will need to evaluate you in the clinic or office. If these symptoms arise after hours, you may be directed to the emergency room in a local hospital. As part of this evaluation, the blood cell counts will be measured. If the white blood cell counts are low, additional tests, such as blood and urine cultures, will be obtained and a chest X-ray ordered. If the source of infection is found, you will be treated accordingly. You will most likely receive antibiotic treatment, either orally or by intravenous injection. If the infection is more severe and intravenous antibiotics are required, you may be admitted to the hospital for the treatment and observation.

In addition to frequent hand washing and avoidance of sick person contact, other steps to decrease risk of infection include: bathing or showering daily using mild soaps; using care when trimming nails; avoiding enemas or suppositories; cooking food fully; washing fruits and vegetables before eating; avoiding cleaning cat litter boxes, bird cages, or fish tanks; and treating other health problems promptly and adequately.

MOUTH SORES

Some patients develop mouth sores during the second week of chemotherapy. If you receive radiation therapy along with chemotherapy, you may experience more severe toxicity. Painful ulcers can interfere with eating and swallowing, so you should keep your mouth clean by gentle brushing of teeth and rinsing after each meal. Use of over-the-counter mouthwash or prescription mouthwash is recommended. However it is important to note that you should not use mouthwash that contains alcohol as this can cause further irritation. Local pain reliever or oral pain pills may be required. If there are thick white or cream-colored spots in your mouth, you should inform a doctor or nurse right away, as these may be signs of oral thrush (a yeast infection).

FATIGUE

Fatigue often occurs after the surgery and also during radiation therapy and chemotherapy. You will feel tired and lack energy to perform activities of daily living, and this can be a variable but often distressing experience. Many factors may impact the severity of fatigue. Anemia can cause or exacerbate fatigue and insufficient food intake due to lack of appetite or nausea/vomiting is another reason. However, for most patients, the exact cause of fatigue is unclear. Correction of a possible cause of fatigue such as anemia or nutritional deficiency may be necessary. Physical therapy, stress management, relaxation, and other psychosocial interventions can be helpful. Frequent exercise such as a brisk walk may help to alleviate some of the fatigue caused by treatment.

SIDE EFFECTS ON THE NERVOUS SYSTEM

You may experience taste changes during chemotherapy, and some chemotherapy medications can cause tingling or numbness in the hands and feet, a condition called peripheral neuropathy. This side effect is usually temporary, but can be permanent in a small number of patients. Your doctor will evaluate and monitor this problem throughout the treatment and afterwards. Chemotherapy can also affect the brain. Perhaps you have heard the term "chemo brain." This refers to the cognitive impairment that some cancer patients experience while undergoing chemotherapy treatment. You may complain of memory loss, or an inability to concentrate or perform multiple tasks. These symptoms are usually mild and most resolve fully after chemotherapy. Research is underway to investigate the exact mechanism and cause of this condition.

SIDE EFFECTS ON SEXUAL AND REPRODUCTIVE FUNCTION

Since chemotherapy can cause birth defects, it is important for women of child-bearing age to receive a pregnancy test and discuss birth control before starting treatment. Some chemotherapy drugs can affect ovarian function and hormone levels in the body. Women may experience irregular periods or even premature menopause as a result of cancer treatment. Some women may be unable to become pregnant after receiving chemotherapy. The oncologist can refer a patient (male or female) to a fertility specialist to discuss options of pursuing fertility. Some patients may experience a decrease in sexual desire. For instance, some male patients may be unable to develop an erection while on treatment, but there are medicines that can help men who have erectile dysfunction.

TARGETED THERAPY

New targeted therapy may be given alone or in combination with chemotherapy. Usually these treatments are well tolerated if patients do not have conditions that prohibit their use. Side effects of Avastin include high blood pressure (hypertension), protein loss in the urine (proteinuria), coughing up blood (hemoptysis), or bleeding. Side effects of Tarceva and other oral medications include skin rash, dry skin, diarrhea, or shortness of breath. Side effects of Erbitux include allergic reactions, skin rash, dry skin, constipation, fatigue, weakness, or abdominal pain. These side effects are manageable with standard medical treatment. For patients with high blood pressure, medications for hypertension will be used to lower the blood pressure. For skin rashes, a steroid or antibacterial cream/lotion may be prescribed. Side effects usually go away after the treatment is over.

SUMMARY

Side effects can occur as a result of any type of lung cancer treatment. It is important for you to be well informed before initiating treatment. You should not hesitate to talk to your cancer care team about any concerns or fears. This is a critical time if you are facing lung cancer because you need both professional support and strong support from your loved ones. With careful monitoring and better supportive care, most side effects can be managed to ensure the completion of cancer treatment while preserving your best quality of life.

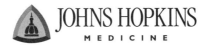

CHAPTER 5

STRAIGHT TALK— COMMUNICATION WITH FAMILY, FRIENDS, AND COWORKERS

DONALD LIST, MSW, LCSW-C; CAROLE SEDDON, MA, LCSW-C, BCD, OSW-C; AND JUSTIN F. KLAMERUS, MD

The phrase "I have cancer" carries tremendous meaning and emotion for any person who must disclose this reality. Communication related to the diagnosis of lung cancer is challenging for patients and their loved ones for countless reasons, but honest, compassionate, age-appropriate communication is essential for anyone coping with this disease. Our hope is that this chapter will help you and your loved ones to talk honestly and openly about cancer.

COMMUNICATION WITH CHILDREN

Parents and caregivers believe that one of their most important responsibilities in life is to protect their children from harm, both physical and emotional. Understandably, many parents who have been diagnosed with cancer find it extraordinarily difficult to tell their children and teenagers about their cancer. In fact, explaining a serious illness can often be one of the most difficult and emotional things you, as a parent, can do.

Parents often share with healthcare professionals that one of their greatest concerns and fears is how their disease and its treatment will affect their children. Some wonder "IF" they should tell their children and may feel completely ill-equipped to have this kind of discussion. In many instances, a patient and parent's main priority is to limit both the short- and long-term effects of cancer treatment on his/her sons and daughters.

As the first step in this process, you may worry about how to tell your children what has happened. As a parent, you have nurtured your children and exposed them to the many wonderful things in life—values, love, honesty, and compassion, among others, and having to talk to them about your illness most likely catches you off guard.

It is understandable for you to feel somewhat bewildered about whether, when, or how to share this information with your children and adolescents. We'd like to share with you what professionals think are important points to consider in assisting you and your children to cope and adjust as healthily as possible as you begin this journey together.

WHY SHOULD I TELL MY CHILDREN?

All illness causes disruption in a family's life. There may be multiple doctor appointments, hospital visits for treatment, and/or hospital admissions. Children and adolescents are amazingly intuitive creatures. They know when something is upsetting or worrying a parent or caregiver. Children and teens thrive on routine—it helps them feel safe. When life becomes unpredictable, they need help adjusting to the changes. The guiding principle should *always* be to *tell the truth* in such a way that one's children are able to understand and prepare themselves for the changes that will occur in family life while mom or dad or another family member is sick. Remember that sometimes a child's question doesn't make sense, or raises enormous topics that you may not know how to address. Tease out exactly what your child wants to know. If children are not told by a parent or loved one, they will, without a doubt, hear about the illness from another, perhaps a classmate, friend, or neighbor. Understandably, finding out about your illness in this manner would provide your children with potentially wrong or misleading information that may very well add to their anxiety.

Not talking to your children may also give them the message that it is not okay to talk about your illness. It becomes the "deep, dark family secret" that no one has permission to speak about. It is common knowledge that children have very active imaginations, and they will use their imagination to come to conclusions about questions that they may feel they cannot ask or talk about. Often this may lead to self-blame or to inaccurate conclusions as to what has happened to a parent or caregiver. This may provoke more angst than the actual truth.

HOW DO I TELL MY CHILDREN?

Facilitating honest communication and age-appropriate understanding is extremely important to help children cope with a parent's serious illness. The more painful a new event is, the more important it is to talk about it with your kids. Children in a family need the right information since those outside of the family may have the wrong information. Open and honest communication should also seek to provide comfort and hope that the family will get through the illness together. It is okay if your discussions don't go perfectly; remember, it is better to have a "bad" talk about things than to not talk about them at all.

Talk to your children about what is happening as soon as you have a good appreciation of your medical situation and are comfortable with the information you've obtained from your medical team.

It is important to consider your children's ages when deciding what and how much you should tell them about your diagnosis. Children and adolescents are inclined to cope more healthily when they are provided with all the information about your cancer at their level of understanding. It's best if children and teens hear what is happening in the family from those who love them and from those they trust. They are a part of the family, and as such, they will be a part of the experience that the illness has on the daily life of the family.

As we know, children will take their cues from their parents and act accordingly. An effective way to get children to talk about their feelings is for parents to express their own feelings. Share your feelings with your children; it models and normalizes appropriate emotional responses in dealing with serious illness. The more you talk to them and include them in things that are happening, the less vulnerable and afraid they will feel.

Many parents are reluctant to use the word "cancer," preferring to use euphemisms such as "lump" or "boo-boo." The parents worry that the word "cancer" may sound too scary to their child. However, euphemisms often lead to confusion and anxiety. They can convey the frightening notion that any "lump" or "boo-boo," including the usual scraped knees and elbows, might mean the beginning of a serious or life-threatening illness for the child.

Parents or caregivers should provide children the opportunity to ask questions and express their feelings. If they ask questions you can't answer, tell them you don't know. You might explain to them that their question is a very good one but "I just don't know the answer." Promise to speak to the doctor and get the answers to their questions.

Additionally, it is helpful to explore the "real" question that the child is trying to ask. "What got you wondering about that?" or "What part did you want to know about?" will help parents understand the child's underlying question or concern. You should be prepared to repeat information multiple times if needed.

If at all possible, both parents should talk to the children. A single parent might ask a close relative or friend to be a part of this discussion. A doctor, nurse, or social worker can also help with difficult discussions. It's helpful to choose a good time to talk, when you are feeling calm. It will be a great help to your child if you can be as calm and objective as possible when you discuss cancer, especially if you are the one who is ill. Some parents find it useful to write down what it is they want to tell their children before they have the discussion with them. It's also helpful to practice the conversation with your partner or a close relative before you talk with your children. Many patients tell us that this makes them feel more comfortable. Explain to your children how their lives might change. Children and teens thrive on routines. Since cancer treatment can disrupt those routines, it is important to prepare them for possible changes to school, chores, or other activities. It is also very important that you prepare your children for the possible effects of treatment. Cancer and cancer treatment can often affect one's appearance. Physical changes such as hair or weight loss can sometimes cause children to think a parent or loved one has changed, that they are somehow different. It is best to explain this to children beforehand so they are prepared. Seeing a father bald does not traumatize a child if they know that that's an expected side effect of chemo. For example, you might say, "When daddy was sick in the hospital, he lost weight, and his hair fell out—but don't worry, it will grow back. He is still the same daddy on the inside."

Lastly, allow your children to participate in your care by understanding your treatment. Give them age-appropriate tasks allowing for demystification of the treatment process. They can think that a situation is worse than it really is. Encourage them to accompany you to the hospital for treatment when possible. As much as you are able, make communicating with your children a priority. Treatment may sap your strength, leaving you with less energy, but make every effort to really listen to your children. This will show them how much you love them, and will help them to feel comfortable coming to you with their concerns in the future. As always, show your children a lot of love and affection. Let them know that although things are different now, your love for them will never change.

In the following sections are some helpful hints and strategies for communicating with children at various developmental stages.

Preschool- and Kindergarten-Age Children (3–5 Years)

Children from 3 to 5 years of age react mostly to their feelings as opposed to facts. Developmentally, they feel like life revolves around them. They are beginning to understand the difference between being well and sick. They engage in magical thinking, thinking that wishing or hoping or even having angry thoughts can make something happen. So it makes sense that preschoolers may worry that they caused their parent to be sick with cancer. It is important to explain and reinforce that they did not do anything to cause the illness of the loved one. Provide brief and simple explanations. Assure them that they cannot "catch" cancer, like a cold or chicken pox. Listen and be alert to their feelings, which they may express through speech or play. Reassure them that they will be taken care of and will not be forgotten. Continue to discipline your children and to set limits for improper behavior. Encourage them to have fun at school or participate in activities that bring them joy and stimulation.

Primary School-Age Children (6–12 Years)

Children in this age group are able to understand more complex explanations of cancer, and they can generally understand basic information about cancer cells. Your disclosure to them may help to fill in gaps in their understanding and knowledge about the disease. It is best to be up-front with them and to provide honest and accurate information about your lung cancer. If they detect that you are shielding them from the truth, this could jeopardize their trust in you. They may feel guilty about things they've said or done to the sick parent. Assure them that their behavior or thoughts did not cause your cancer. Take time to listen to them and to make certain that they know you care about their feelings. Reassure them about their care and your plans to help them maintain their schedule and routine as much as is possible. Have patience; children at this age still think the world revolves around them most of the time. This kind of thinking, more often than not, does not change when there are difficulties in the family such as a serious illness. Don't be surprised if they don't seem to understand what the sick parent is going through. Be patient. Try not to make them feel guilty for wanting to go on with their normal routines (sports, school or church activities, or fun times with their friends). Routine is important to children because it makes them feel secure and safe.

Teenagers (13–18 Years)

Teenagers are unpredictable! Teenagers need to know the truth and may feel particularly hurt by information that they feel is incomplete or inaccurate. You might communicate to them something like "I'm telling you all that I know right now. If anything changes, I promise I will tell you." Appreciate that there are a range of potential responses teenagers may have. Be mindful that teenagers are often uncomfortable with some of their thoughts and feelings. Teenagers are able to begin thinking more like adults and many desire detailed information about a parent's illness. They may feel an overwhelming sense of responsibility to become more involved that conflicts with their need for their own independence, and this may cause guilt or frustration. They may worry about their parent, but may hide this worry by avoiding the discussion or absorbing themselves in an activity outside of the family. Teenagers struggle with the need for independence, and a parent's illness may make this more difficult. Encourage your teenager to spend time with friends in age-appropriate activities. Most teens also crave privacy. They may or may not want to talk about the experience with their family. The teen's relationships outside of family are so very important. Encourage your teenagers to seek support from other sources, like an aunt, a friend's parent, a teacher, or another member of the extended family.

IS MOMMY GOING TO DIE?

If you are concerned about discussing death with your children, you're not alone. Many of us hesitate to talk about death, particularly with children. But death is an inescapable fact of life. We have no choice but to deal with it and so must our children; if we are to help them, we must let them know it is okay to talk about death. By talking to children about death, we discover what they know (and don't know) and their fears, misconceptions, and worries. Through open and honest discussions, we can then help them by providing them with information, comfort, and understanding. The basic questions about life and death demand honest answers.

Listen carefully when children ask questions. Make sure you understand what they want to know. Honestly answer the questions. If your child asks "Am I going to die?", tell him or her that everyone dies, but hopefully that will not be for a long time. If a child asks whether a parent is going to die, again explain that all people die eventually, but hopefully mom or dad won't die for a long time. If the family practices a religious tradition, parents often use this opportunity to explain their religion's teaching on death and afterlife. Perhaps your place of worship has individuals with training and expertise in these areas. A child may ask a question that a parent cannot answer. It is honest and okay to say "I don't know." Children need time to absorb the news. Don't expect perfection—from children or yourself. There is no "perfect" way to have this conversation.

COMMUNICATION WITH COWORKERS AND FRIENDS

"A real friend is one who walks in when the rest of the world walks out."

—Walter Winchell, famous columnist

Those of us who work with cancer patients have a unique vantage point on how the lives of our patients are influenced and changed by this disease. One miracle that is seen again and again is the gift that love and friendship bestows on many of our patients afflicted with cancer. Our hope is that every cancer patient knows the healing comfort of friendship.

Just as disclosing the diagnosis of lung cancer to children is painful and challenging, so too is sharing this news with our friends and coworkers. For many of us, our health conditions can be quite private matters. We often only share these conditions with our closest friends and family. Cancer patients may feel the same way during the initial portion of their illness. This is natural. If you are the patient with lung cancer, we recommend sharing the news of your diagnosis with your key friends and allies slowly, and in a manner that feels comfortable to you. These individuals can be a source of comfort and support in unimaginable ways.

Along with concerns over privacy, some patients are concerned to reveal that they have cancer to coworkers, as they feel that this will show vulnerability. You are not required to tell your boss or coworkers that you have cancer—simply that you are under doctor's care that will require time away from work. In the past, your health issues may never have been discussed at work, but with cancer, we suggest an open discussion with those at work. This may be limited to your direct supervisor and human resources staff, or if you feel comfortable, a more open disclosure with other co-workers. Having these discussions early on in the journey through cancer diagnosis and treatment may help to give you peace of mind about your job.

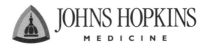

CHAPTER 6

MAINTAINING BALANCE—
WORK AND LIFE DURING
TREATMENT

DONALD LIST, MSW-C, LCSW-C; CAROLE
SEDDON, MA, LCSW-C, BCD, OSW-C;
AND JUSTIN F. KLAMERUS, MD

Navigating the complexities of cancer treatment and managing the side effects of cancer therapy can be a tall order. Patients, often used to a fast-paced life, find it difficult to adjust to these new challenges and maintain balance in life. This is common.

In the first chapter, we described the common experience of shock and immobility following the diagnosis of lung cancer. Although those initial days are often filled with distress and fear, the days that follow can be trying in many other ways—including having to face the pressures of incoming medical bills, to make key decisions about returning to work and in what capacity, to acknowledge and accept the new limitations on one's health, and sadly, for some patients, to understand that the time to live may be limited. Each of these issues and myriad other challenges facing lung cancer patients would be enough to cripple the strongest person. Yet, for those of us given the privilege of caring for these patients, we have seen a wondrous strength and resounding courage in so many of our patients. This spirit can be a force to face any hurdle, especially when it is supported by loving and caring friends and family.

PRIORITIES

One of the key ingredients to maintaining balance is an understanding of what is most important. In his book, *Seven Habits of Highly Effective People*, the legendary success consultant Dr. Stephen Covey describes this process so well when he says that highly effective people work diligently to "put first things first" in their personal and professional lives. A helpful exercise for you as a lung cancer patient is to make the same assessment of what is most important in your personal and work lives.

Using the model described by Dr. Covey, imagine all of the roles you have in your life: parent, spouse, child, friend, corporate lawyer, community volunteer, and even patient. Define what is most important to you in each of these roles. Perhaps some are less important when balancing a cancer diagnosis and facing treatment. That's okay. The purpose is to articulate what your "main things" are in life and to make future decisions based on this understanding. In addition to identifying the important roles in your life, it is also helpful to plan for the tasks and duties associated with each important role. For instance, you might list attending your daughter's wedding next month as a highly important task in your role as a parent. Because this is such a significant priority, you may need to change a scheduled chemotherapy appointment so that treatment doesn't interfere with this important priority and role.

Each of us commonly makes decisions like these in our daily lives. The more stressed or limited we are in terms of time, the more important it is to define our priorities. From watching hundreds of cancer patients, we believe that the patients who understand their priorities are the ones who face cancer with greater balance and control.

NAVIGATING WORK AND PROFESSIONAL RESPONSIBILITIES

Many cancer patients who are physically able to work, continue working in some capacity during their treatments. Work is an important source of fulfillment for many of us and we take seriously the responsibilities that we have in our work lives. If you choose to work, you must make conscious efforts to balance the priorities of your health with the real-world realities of work. If you must take a medical leave-of-absence, you may be eager to return to work as soon as it is safe for you to do so. Returning to work usually helps cancer patients to feel some sense that they are getting their lives back. This can be quite emotionally satisfying and very helpful for healing. In addition to these psychological benefits, an important factor for many patients is the ongoing need for the salary and benefits that their work provides, including health insurance.

If you plan to work through treatment, we suggest asking each of your doctors and other medical providers for a detailed description of your treatment plan. If you are receiving radiation, don't be afraid to ask the radiation department for an appointment time that accommodates your work schedule with as minimal an interruption as possible. Most radiation appointments can be given on the same time each weekday. If you are on chemotherapy, we suggest requesting a schedule of all appointments for each cycle of treatment. In most instances, this will allow you the opportunity to make plans for this 3 to 4 week period. Once these appointments are known, share them with your employer. However, both you and your employer must realize that cancer treatment will require flexibility.

Early in treatment, we also encourage patients to have frank discussions with their physicians and nurses as to how the treatment will affect them in their personal and professional lives. For instance, some forms of cancer therapy may weaken your immune system and you may not be able to be around large numbers of people without certain precautions. In addition, you may feel fatigued from treatments and find it difficult to keep up with your personal and professional responsibilities with the same endurance as you did prior to treatment. This may mean asking your employer to change some of your job responsibilities and expectations.

If it becomes necessary to take a leave-of-absence, you should speak with the appropriate human resources personnel as soon as possible to find out what benefits are available to you, such as personal sick leave, short and long-term disability, or even banked sick time given by fellow employees. Although you might have short and/or long-term disability coverage, it is also crucial to know exactly how much pay you will be receiving while on disability benefits. The financial costs related to cancer treatment can mean significant changes for many families. If your job does not provide sick time or paid leave, it is important to note that you and your family may receive benefits from the Family and Medical Leave Act (FMLA).

Coworkers often bank their unused sick leave to share with cancer patients receiving aggressive and extended care.

There are important issues to consider. For example, the use of shared sick leave requires that colleagues must know that you are seriously ill and that you will be out of work for an extended period of time. Also, colleagues must be willing to give away their own protected sick leave benefits. Many patients are private with their personal health matters and utilizing this shared benefit often means considerable disclosure. It is also worth noting that most of our patients describe the support that they receive from colleagues at work as a source of significant comfort through the challenges of their cancer journey.

Once treatment begins, it is important that your employer or supervisor receive periodic updates from you. Many employers will require that paperwork describing treatments and the resulting limitations on work be completed by your treating physician(s). Allow ample time for completion of these documents by requesting them from treating physicians as soon as possible.

Many cancer patients find colleagues at work to be very supportive and caring. For others, unfortunately, their places of employment are not supportive. Sadly, many case managers and social workers who work with oncology patients report not infrequently that some employers believe that they have to let an employee go as soon as they are told that the employee has cancer. In many cases, this is unlawful.

Four federal laws provide some job protection to cancer patients: the *Americans with Disabilities Act (ADA)*, the *Federal Rehabilitation Act*, the *Family and Medical Leave Act*, and the *Employee Retirement and Income Security Act*.

The ADA was enacted to cover U.S. citizens who are disabled. Coverage by the ADA is determined on a case-by-case basis. In terms of finding a job, under this act, a prospective employer may not ask a prospective employee if they have ever had cancer. An employer has the right to know only if the employee is able to do the work required by the job being offered. For more information, contact the ADA, Disability and Technical Assistance Center at (800) 949-4232.

Prior to the Americans with Disabilities Act in 1990, the Federal Rehabilitation Act was the only federal law that prohibited cancer-based employment discrimination. The Rehabilitation Act bans public employers and private employers who receive public funds from discriminating on the basis of a disability. For more information, contact their office at (888) 37-OFCCP.

In 1993, Congress enacted the Family and Medical Leave Act to provide job security to workers who must attend to the serious medical needs of themselves or their family members. This act requires covered employers to provide up to 12 weeks of unpaid, job-protected leave for family members who need time off to address their own serious illness or to care for a seriously ill child, parent, spouse, or healthy newborn or newly adopted child. Although this legislation was a significant leap forward to protect workers, there are significant limitations. For more information please call the National Partnership for Women & Families at (202) 986-2600.

The Employee Retirement and Income Security Act (ERISA) prohibits any employer from discriminating against an employee for the purpose of preventing him or her from collecting benefits under an employee benefit plan. All employers who offer benefit packages to their employees are subject to ERISA. Information about ERISA can be obtained at http://www.dol.gov/dol/topic/health -plans/erisa.htm.

We recommend that you contact the social worker provided by your local hospital or treatment center if you are struggling with employment or benefit issues. These professionals have experience in navigating many of these struggles and may be able to direct you to additional resources to help you through your treatment.

NAVIGATING HEALTH ISSUES

As Chapter 4 outlines, many of the side effects of therapy can be anticipated and minimized by the advances in supportive care. Balancing the health challenges brought about by cancer and cancer treatment will require close communication between you and your treatment team.

All cancer patients should have available to them the contact information for their treating physicians and support staff assisting them with patient care. When new symptoms arise, inform these individuals as soon as possible.

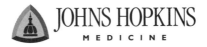

CHAPTER 7

SURVIVING LUNG CANCER—
RE-ENGAGING IN MIND
AND BODY HEALTH AFTER
TREATMENT

AMY E. DEZERN, MD; AND JUSTIN F.
KLAMERUS, MD

Kathlyn Conway, in her excellent book *Ordinary Life: A Memoir of Illness*, writes "Cancer has become only a piece of the quilt that is my life. In looking at the piece as part of the whole quilt, I can view it from different angles, in different light, in relation to all the other pieces. My present task is to take the broader view, to regain a sense of the fullness of my life....The hard task for me and my family is to integrate each of our experiences of cancer into who we are."

So far in this book, we have guided you through the process of dealing with much of the physical and day-to-day needs of a patient facing lung cancer treatment. We've discussed diagnosis, treatment, side effects, and even how to navigate difficult decisions during this challenging time. We would be grossly negligent if we did not provide a discussion of the "mind-body connections" that many of our cancer patients face during their illnesses. For many patients with lung cancer, this may include anxiety, depression, insomnia, fatigue, and other distressing feelings and emotions. Just like the pieces of the quilt that composed the author's view of her illness, the emotional aspects of cancer are very real and need proper attention. In the final section of this chapter we will explore the issues concerning survivorship and how to approach the completion of therapy.

SURVIVING CANCER EMOTIONALLY

A very famous myth in Greek mythology is the story of Pandora. As the legend goes, Zeus created Pandora as punishment for mankind. At the time of her creation, Pandora was given a large box by Zeus and told to keep it closed. Unfortunately, Pandora was also given the gift of curiosity, which led her to eventually open the large box. When she opened the box, evils, ills, disease, and burdensome labor befell the earth. The story of Pandora is one that many cancer patients describe to us—their journey through cancer has been like "opening Pandora's box" in their life. Once the box was opened, it couldn't be closed again. For many patients this means facing the realities of serious illness, limitations in physical wellness, and maybe even facing one's own mortality. All of these challenges affect our emotions; this is natural. We encourage you to explore your feelings with family members, close friends, and other sources of support that might be important to you. In particular, if you or your loved one has a history of mental illness such as depression, anxiety, or substance abuse, we encourage you to talk with a mental health professional as part of your comprehensive treatment plan.

ANXIETY

Facing cancer diagnosis and treatment is likely to cause a significant amount of stress for you and your family. In fact, anxiety is one of the most common responses that our patients describe following this news. Numerous studies have shown that up to 50% of cancer patients suffer from anxiety during their cancer illness. Anxiety is a feeling of unease, fear, or the sense of impending harm or distress. The feelings are usually accompanied by heightened arousal or worry in reaction to real or perceived threats to your well-being.

Along with the mental and emotional feelings that accompany anxiety, physical signs and symptoms may occur as well. Common signs and symptoms include sweating, fast breathing, shortness of breath, palpitations (heart skipping beats), and tremor (trembling hands). You may also experience difficulty with concentration, poor sleep quality/duration (insomnia), restlessness, and muscle tension.

Although many patients experience these symptoms during their journey, an important question is how disabling or incapacitating these symptoms are for the patient. We encourage you to discuss these symptoms as early on in treatment as possible. Anxiety and other mood disorders such as depression have a very negative impact on the patient's quality of life. If your symptoms are severe or disabling, your doctor or mental health professional may suggest treatment.

Many successful treatments are available for patients who suffer from anxiety. One of the most important considerations is to make certain that your treatment plan is individualized. You are the patient and all therapies should be tailored to your specific needs. Avoid taking medications that aren't prescribed for you and be very mindful of the dangers of using drugs or alcohol to relieve psychological symptoms.

There are two broad categories of therapy for patients afflicted with anxiety: behavioral and pharmacologic. In general, neither modality will work without the other. We encourage patients to receive education from their nurses, physicians, and mental health professionals about the symptoms that they are experiencing and how they are best managed. Social support (such as that which is available from family, friends, spiritual leaders, and cancer support groups) is an excellent source of comfort for cancer patients who are experiencing anxiety. One particular program, entitled "I Can Cope," is sponsored by the American Cancer Society. Many patients also benefit from professional therapy offered by a social worker, psychologist, or psychiatrist who has expertise in the mental health needs of cancer patients.

Growing data also supports the use of relaxation, guided imagery, music therapy, and other complementary therapies, such as acupuncture and massage, to treat anxiety associated with serious illness. Increasingly, patients are utilizing herbal supplements to treat medical conditions. We strongly discourage the use of these agents while you are undergoing treatment. Many of these agents can have serious drug interactions with chemotherapeutic agents. If you are using an herbal remedy, please make your healthcare team aware of all of these agents and do not begin use without prior discussion with your healthcare team.

The pharmacologic management of anxiety focuses on a class of drugs called benzodiazepines (Table 2). The most common side effect of this class of medications is sedation or the sense of feeling tired. Patients do often accommodate to these symptoms and the sleepiness gradually subsides. As with any new medication, be sure to discuss all side effects with your doctor or pharmacist. Elderly patients should be particularly cautious when starting a drug in this class. Older patients may experience heightened anxiety, delirium, disorientation, or even problems walking following treatment with benzodiazepines. Once a patient has started taking benzodiazepines on a regular basis, they should not abruptly stop these medicines. A withdrawal syndrome can occur with discontinuation of any of these drugs.

Table 2 Benzodiazepines Available in the United States

Drug	Trade Name	Usual Dose Range (mg/day)	Comments
Chlordiazepoxide	Librium	15–100 mg	Long-acting
Diazepam	Valium	2–40 mg	Long-acting with rapid oral absorption
Oxazepam	Serax	30–120 mg	Short-acting
Lorazepam	Ativan	2–6 mg	Short-acting
Alprazolam	Xanax	0.5–6.0 mg	Short-acting

DEPRESSION

Depression and other mood disorders are very common in patients with cancer. When patients describe feeling "depressed" they often express a sense of despair, gloominess, sadness, unhappiness, or heaviness of heart. Experiencing these symptoms is not necessarily a sign of mental illness. Most individuals experience feelings such as these while undergoing the normal grief response that is brought on by facing a major illness and these symptoms should begin to improve or resolve within a few weeks. A respected study exploring the incidence of mood disorders and mental illness in cancer patients found that most patients suffer from an *adjustment disorder* and not *major depression*. Adjustment disorders occur when psychological stressors, such as facing a major illness like lung cancer, leads to significant behavioral and emotional symptoms. As with anxiety, depressed mood, adjustment disorder, and major depression occur on a continuum. Prompt recognition and attention to these symptoms can significantly improve quality of life.

Several studies have developed screening questions to assess depression in cancer patients. Two of the most helpful questions are:

1. Are you depressed most of the day, nearly every day?

2. Are you bothered by loss of interest in all or almost all activities?

These questions correctly identify depressed and non-depressed individuals. If you or your loved one answers yes to either of these questions, please speak with your healthcare professional to consider treatment for depression.

There are many risk factors that increase the likelihood of development of depression in patients with lung cancer. These include younger age (due to less experience adapting to illness and physical limitations), poorer health status (more advanced stage of lung cancer, unrelieved symptoms, etc.), history of mental illness before the cancer diagnosis, treatment failure, or recurrence of cancer. In addition, many medications can cause depressed mood as a side effect. You may be at particular risk depending on the serious nature of your diagnosis, the loss of functional status that may result from the disease, and the fact that many patients present with advanced disease with a limited chance of cure.

There are many effective therapeutic approaches to treatment of depressed mood, adjustment disorder, and depression. A thorough evaluation and assessment by a mental health professional is encouraged for patients who experience severe symptoms.

As with treatment for anxiety, the treatment of mood disorders falls into two broad categories: cognitive/behavioral and pharmacologic. With respect to cognitive and behavioral treatment, the most effective management comes from consistent emotional support. For many patients, this emotional support can come from family, friends, and other forms of social support. Cancer support groups are particularly helpful and many studies have identified that support group participation results in sustained improvement in symptoms of depression, anxiety, and healthy social functioning. Two excellent resources for more information include the American Cancer Society and Cancer*Care*.

For some patients, emotional support is best provided by a mental health professional. Whenever possible, we encourage patients and their families to meet with an oncology social worker to discuss options in their communities. Counseling services are provided by licensed social workers, psychologists, and psychiatrists. Formal psychotherapy is often only provided by psychologists and psychiatrists.

Many prescription medications are approved for the treatment of depression and most are safe to use in patients with cancer. Medications to treat depression affect key chemical signaling pathways in the brain that are thought

to be disturbed by depression. The most commonly prescribed antidepressants belong to a class of medications
known as selective serotonin reuptake inhibitors (SSRIs)
(see Table 3). SSRIs may cause nausea, dry mouth, headache, nervousness, drowsiness, loss of sex drive, and even
low blood pressure. Newer drugs in this class are generally
better tolerated by our patients.

Table 3 Selective Serotonin Reuptake Inhibitors
Available in the United States

Drug	Trade Name	Usual Dose Range (mg/day)	Comments
Citaloproam	Celexa	10–40 mg	
Escitalopram	Lexapro	5–20 mg	Newer SSRI with fewer side effects
Fluoxetine	Prozac	10–40 mg	
Fluvoxamine	Luvox	25–100 mg	
Paroxetine	Paxil	10–50 mg	May cause significant nausea
Sertraline	Zoloft	50–200 mg	

Other drugs commonly used to treat depression include:
Wellbutrin (bupropion), Effexor (venlafaxine), Serzone (ne-
fazodone), and Remeron (mirtazapine). Remeron can be
a good antidepressant for cancer patients who are losing
weight because one of the side effects of this agent is increased appetite and resultant weight gain.

There are three important considerations to remember
when starting antidepressant therapy:

1. Many prescription treatments for depression take several weeks to become effective and patients should not

expect immediate improvement in depressive symptoms upon starting an antidepressant.

2. The FDA warns that all patients taking antidepressants should be monitored closely for worsening symptoms of depression and suicidal thoughts. This is uncommon but has been reported for these medicines.

3. The recommended starting doses of antidepressants in cancer patients are lower than other healthy patients. In addition, dose escalation should occur slowly. Patients and their healthcare providers must monitor patients closely for side effects.

Cancer patients often talk with their oncologists and nurses about *attitude*. A positive attitude is an important tool for patients to use against cancer. When examining many studies on quality of life and survival, patients who are able to keep a positive attitude often fare better than those who have a negative attitude. This is certainly easier said than done, and if you are feeling down, you can't wish that away. What you can do is reach out to your sources of support and ask for help. Talking with other patients who have completed treatment for cancer is particularly helpful for many patients. The Anderson Network through MD Anderson Cancer Center is a great patient-to-patient support network that can be accessed over the phone. We encourage all patients and their families to find a local support group to help with this process.

Also, remember that experiencing the symptoms described above may also be related to the treatments for your cancer. These can include prescription drug side effects (for example, steroids used to treat nausea or as a pre-medication before chemotherapy can cause or heighten symptoms of anxiety), the effects of uncontrolled pain, or an abnormal metabolic state within the body (such as high calcium or low sodium blood levels) could mimic depression. Please explain all symptoms to your healthcare provider so they may be investigated fully.

CANCER SURVIVORSHIP—MOVING FORWARD

Cancer survivor—this is a term we hear often as more and more people are living with, through, and beyond cancer. There are more than 10 million cancer survivors in the United States today, and millions more who, as family members and friends of cancer patients, have been touched by the disease. As you move forward after your treatment ends, you may be slightly altered on both the inside and outside by the impact that lung cancer has had on your life. While those around you are celebrating the completion of your treatment, you may be left with a number of unexpected emotional, physical, and practical issues.

Few things are more exciting for a cancer patient than when that last IV is taken out, the scan looks good, and no more chemotherapy or radiation is planned. This is a milestone to be celebrated. It is important to note that, even when not receiving therapy, many patients are affected by the physical and emotional reminders of their therapy. Late effects can be the side effects, complications, or adverse outcomes that are persistent and are the result of the disease process, the treatment, or both.

One to five percent of patients who lost their hair from their chemotherapy may never grow it back as it was before. Cardiac toxicities from the radiation to the lungs can cause symptoms of heart failure years later. Neuropathy (numbness and tingling pain) or sensorineural hearing loss from Platinol-AQ may never completely resolve, requiring additional medication to manage the symptoms. During and following chemotherapy, some patients experience difficulties with memory, attention, and other aspects of cognitive function. This constellation of complaints commonly is referred to as "chemo brain." Although the syndrome is not understood completely, as the cancer survival rate improves, it is receiving greater attention from healthcare professionals and researchers.

RESOURCES FOR SURVIVORS

There are many excellent advocacy groups available for cancer survivors. One group in particular, the National Coalition for Cancer Survivorship (NCCS) has a very helpful Web site for cancer survivors at http://www.canceradvocacy. org. The NCCS also publishes *The Cancer Survival Toolbox*, which is a free, self-learning audio program developed by cancer organizations to help people develop important skills to meet and understand the challenges of their cancer diagnosis. The toolbox contains a set of basic skills to help navigate diagnosis, and special topics on key issues faced by people with cancer. See Chapter 11 for more information about this and other resources.

SUMMARY

Although it may seem that facing cancer has been analogous to "opening Pandora's box," you and your support network will gather the resources and strength to face the challenges ahead. It's worth going back to the myth of Pandora for a moment because, just as disease and hardship escaped from the box and challenged the people, at the very bottom of Pandora's box lay hope. With the proper supports around you, including this guide, we anticipate that you will find the hope that you need to face this difficult and challenging disease.

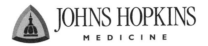

CHAPTER 8

JOHNS HOPKINS
M E D I C I N E

MANAGING RISK—
WHAT IF MY CANCER
COMES BACK?

CHRISTINE HANN, MD, PhD

As described in the previous chapters, cancer therapy may involve surgery, radiation, chemotherapy, or a combination of these treatments. The schedule during many of these treatments tends to be time consuming and demanding. At the completion of treatment, if your cancer has responded to treatment, you may be in complete remission, where no tumor can be detected, or in partial remission, where your tumor has decreased in size but can still be seen. If you are in remission, you will be given a plan of follow-up care to monitor your recovery and to watch closely for any cancer regrowth.

While the goal of cancer therapy is to remove all cancer cells from the body, the likelihood of lung cancer returning depends on many factors, including the type of lung cancer, the stage of cancer you presented with, the treatment you received, and your response to therapy. If the cancer returns, this is called a recurrence and it is usually due to cancer cells that remained in your body after initial treatment. With time, these cells could grow again into a new tumor. When the cancer recurs at or near the original cancer site, it is considered a local recurrence. When the cancer has spread to other organs or sites far away from the original cancer, it is termed a distant recurrence and represents a new stage of disease called metastatic cancer. Your follow-up care will be guided, in part, by the likelihood of your cancer returning and will include doctors' visits and laboratory and radiological studies. Often times you may be the first to notice symptoms that indicate that the cancer has returned so it is important that you have open communication with your healthcare providers.

WHAT CAN I DO FOR MYSELF AFTER TREATMENT HAS FINISHED?

There are many things you can do for yourself to maintain a healthy life after therapy. First and foremost, if you haven't stopped smoking, please do so! If you have quit, congratulations! People with lung cancer have a high risk of developing a second lung cancer and persistent smoking increases this risk. For many patients, the diagnosis of lung cancer is enough to make them stop smoking immediately. Other patients continue to smoke, citing the increased stress of their cancer diagnosis as a reason for ongoing smoking. If you are having difficulty with smoking cessation, please talk to your healthcare providers. There are a variety of medications and resources that may be of help to you. The American Cancer Society and the Office of the Surgeon General have great Web sites that offer tips to help smokers quit.

Other changes that help support a healthy lifestyle include eating well, maintaining a healthy weight, and engaging in moderate exercise. Eating well includes choosing healthy (low-fat and low-salt) foods and eating 5–9 servings daily of fruits and vegetables along with whole grains and beans. Nutritional guidelines have been established by the American Cancer Society. If you would like to speak to someone in person, most hospitals and cancer centers have nutritionists on staff that can answer specific questions. In addition to a healthy diet, try to exercise at a moderate level for at least 30 minutes several times a week. Regular exercise can help to reduce anxiety, fatigue, and pain. Exercise has also been show to elevate your mood. It is wise to start slowly and increase your activity, as tolerated, over time. A combination of a healthy diet and regular exercise will also help you maintain a healthy weight and will likely boost your self-esteem.

FOLLOW-UP ONCOLOGY CARE

After the completion of your primary therapy, you will be scheduled for regular visits with your healthcare team. These visits should include review of any symptoms you may be having, a physical exam, and radiologic and laboratory studies. General guidelines recommend follow-up visits every 4–6 months for the first two years and then annually for an additional 3 years. It is common to have scheduled visits at higher frequency—such as every 2–3 months, but this may depend on the type of lung cancer for which you were treated. If, after 5 years of follow-up, you have no evidence of recurrence, you are considered cured and can resume your regularly scheduled health visits to your primary care physician or internist without further visits to your cancer doctors. Despite this, many patients elect to continue seeing their oncologist annually. A commonly asked question is, "Will I need to see all of my doctors for follow-up?" During your primary therapy, you may have received treatment from several doctors and may question whether you need to see all of them in follow-up. Each doctor may want to see you to discuss specific symptoms or side effects you may have had from their particular therapy, such as healing or pain from surgery, or side effects from radiation or chemotherapy. Your doctors, though, should be able to coordinate any laboratory or imaging studies you may need.

WHAT IF MY CANCER COMES BACK?

If your doctors suspect that your cancer has recurred they may send you for more tests including further imaging studies, blood work, or a biopsy. Available treatment modalities include those that may have been used in your original treatment plan such as surgery, radiation, and chemotherapy. If a recurrence is confirmed, your therapy will depend on several factors, including the location of your recurrence, your original treatment, your current health status, and characteristics of your specific tumor. The sections below describe some of the treatment options available.

PATIENTS INITIALLY TREATED FOR LOCALIZED OR EARLY STAGE NSCLC (STAGES I-III)

If you were treated for early stage or localized NSCLC lung cancer your initial treatment should have consisted of surgery or radiation with or without chemotherapy. If you have a local recurrence, your doctors may first want to determine whether the tumor is in a location that can be safely removed by surgery. If it is, and you can tolerate surgery, then that may be a good option. If the tumor cannot be removed safely or you prefer not to undergo surgery, then you may benefit from radiation therapy. As in primary treatments, chemotherapy may also help after surgery or radiation.

If your tumor is in a location that is blocking one of your airways, then local treatments, such as laser therapy, brachytherapy, or photodynamic therapy may be helpful. These are all treatments that treat tumors inside your airways and are performed by pulmonary doctors and radiation oncologists. If your blocked airway is causing significant symptoms, then the pulmonary doctor may also place a stent, or a brace, within your airway to help keep it open and to help you to breathe better.

A distant recurrence occurs when the cancer has spread to other organs or sites far away from the original cancer. Occasionally the cancer may recur at a single distant site, such as the brain or adrenal gland; in these cases, surgery may also be an option. In most cases, distant recurrences occur at several sites and the recommended treatment is chemotherapy. As described in Chapter 3, chemotherapy is a systemic therapy designed to treat cancer in multiple locations. The choices of chemotherapy will depend on the type of therapies you have received in the past and your current health status. Other factors that may be important are the molecular characteristics of your tumor, such as changes in specific proteins, which can be targeted by specific drugs. One example of such a drug is Tarceva, which inhibits the EGFR.

PATIENTS INITIALLY TREATED FOR METASTATIC (STAGE IV) NSCLC

Patients who present with stage IV lung cancer receive combination chemotherapy as first-line therapy. The chance of cure in patients who present with metastatic lung cancer is very low and this stage of cancer is generally considered incurable. For patients with stage IV NSCLC, treatment is focused on controlling symptoms from the cancer and maintaining the best quality of life for the longest time possible. First-line therapy for stage IV lung cancer is presented in the chemotherapy section of Chapter 3. While the rate of cure or complete remission for stage IV lung cancer is low, some patients may have partial responses and stable disease after initial chemotherapy.

Patients whose cancer has recurred after first-line treatment have several options for their next therapies, including second-line therapy, third-line therapy, and beyond. These include chemotherapy, targeted therapy, supportive care, and clinical trials. In general, chemotherapy or targeted therapy is recommended for advanced stages of lung cancer. The choice of therapy will depend on several factors, including characteristics of your tumor, your prior therapy, and your current health status. Local therapies also may be helpful to treat tumors, that have arisen in areas that cause discomfort.

PATIENTS INITIALLY TREATED FOR SCLC

Patients who present with SCLC are initially treated based on the stage of their tumor; those with limited stage SCLC usually receive combination chemotherapy with a platinum drug and Etopophos and radiation to the site of disease. Some limited stage patients can be cured with this regimen. For very small tumors, surgery plus chemotherapy has been successful and is currently being evaluated in clinical trials. Patients diagnosed with more advanced SCLC (extensive stage SCLC) are generally considered incurable and the goal of therapy is to control symptoms and maintain the best quality of life for the longest time possible. In the United States, first-line therapy for SCLC consists of a platinum agent plus Etopophos. In contrast to NSCLC, many patients with SCLC have good responses to chemotherapy including significant tumor shrinkage; some patients will experience complete responses.

Regardless of your initial stage or initial treatment, the recommended therapy for recurrent SCLC is based on the time frame in which the cancer returns. If the cancer recurs after 3 months, then it is considered chemotherapy-sensitive and several chemotherapy regimens are currently recommended. Currently only one drug, Hycamtin, is FDA approved as a second-line agent for chemotherapy-sensitive SCLC.

If the cancer returns shortly after the completion of treatment (<2–3 months), then it is considered resistant to chemotherapy and is termed chemotherapy-refractory SCLC. There is currently no standard treatment for chemotherapy-refractory SCLC. There are several chemotherapy agents that have demonstrated activity in clinical trials that may be used. For most patients with chemotherapy-refractory SCLC, clinical trials may be a very good option.

CLINICAL TRIALS

Clinical trials (see pages 55–58) are not used solely for patients who have exhausted standard therapies. In fact, there are clinical trials designed to be given in the first-line (initial treatment) and second-line (treatment at first recurrence or progression) settings. Successful examples of this approach have been used in lung cancer therapy; for example, the addition of a targeted antibody, Avastin, to standard chemotherapy for metastatic NSCLC improved survival for patients treated in the clinical trial. While the primary benefit of clinical trials is to help develop new therapies for future patients, participation in clinical trials allows some patients access to new treatments to which they would otherwise not have access.

WHAT IF I DON'T WANT OR MY DOCTOR DOESN'T WANT TO GIVE ANY MORE TREATMENT?

As much as patients and their loved ones prepare themselves to receive bad news when seeing their doctors for follow-up, the news of a recurrence is never easy to handle. It is very important to keep an open dialogue with your healthcare providers and to be frank about your feelings regarding therapy and future goals. Some patients may elect to continue on with therapy for as long as they can, while others may feel that further therapy will negatively impact whatever quality of life they may have remaining. In addition your doctor may not want to give you any more treatment. Your doctors should be able to provide you with information on the potential benefits and likely side effects of any therapy to help guide you in this decision. Deciding against further therapy is always a reasonable option but it is a decision that should be born out of frank and detailed conversations with your healthcare providers and loved ones.

If no further anti-cancer therapy is given, other healthcare options are available. Palliative care is focused on minimizing pain and discomfort from cancer. More information on palliative care and hospice are provided in the next chapter. Several forms of therapy, such as radiation therapy that can be delivered to sites of tumor growth where there is pain, are also considered palliative, but are not intended to cure the cancer. Most often, palliative care includes medications to control cancer pain and supplemental oxygen to relieve shortness of breath. Many cancer centers and hospitals have palliative care teams who can provide you with more information and support as you make the adjustment from active therapy to supportive care.

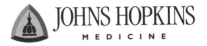

CHAPTER 9

My Cancer Isn't Curable— What Now?

Cynthia Williams, DO, MA; Lynn Billing, RN, CHPN; Justin F. Klamerus, MD; and Julie R. Brahmer, MD, MSc

UNDERSTANDING GOALS OF TREATMENT FOR METASTATIC CANCER

Metastatic cancer occurs when the cancer cells spread from where the cancer started to other parts of your body. Cancer usually spreads through blood vessels and the lymphatic system. When cancer spreads to a different area, the metastatic cancer will be of the same tumor type and will have the same name as the primary tumor (for example, if lung cancer spreads to the liver, it is called "metastatic lung cancer," not liver cancer). The most common sites that lung cancer spreads to are the brain, the liver, and bone. Some people with metastatic cancer do not have any symptoms. Their metastases are found by performing follow-up tests such as X-rays, CT scans, or even blood tests during follow-up visits to their oncologist.

When symptoms of metastatic cancer do occur, the symptom will depend on the area or location where the cancer has spread and the size of the metastasis. For example, cancer that spreads to the bones is likely to cause "achy" pain in the effected bone. In rare instances, a bone fracture may occur for no apparent reason. Cancer that spreads to the brain can cause confusion, headaches, visual changes, weakness in the arms or legs, unsteadiness, or seizures. Abdominal swelling or jaundice (yellowing of the skin) can indicate that cancer has spread to the liver. This is not to say that every new symptom is related to the cancer, but it is always best to notify your doctor if you are having new problems, aches, and pains, or an increase in severity of any symptoms that you have been having.

Treatment of metastatic cancer is focused on controlling the spread of the cancer, decreasing symptoms and improving quality of life, and possibly prolonging life. When cancer has spread, the treatments you and your oncologist will consider will be based on many factors: (1) where the tumor has spread, (2) the size of the tumor, (3) your age, (4) how healthy you are overall, (5) your functional abilities (are you up and about most of the day or do you spend most of your day in bed?), (6) what treatments you have received in the past, and finally (7) what your goals are, what *you* want, and how you feel. Metastatic lung cancer may be treated with chemotherapy, radiation therapy, biological or targeted therapies, or any combination of the above. In addition to these therapies, some patients decide that it is best for them not to receive additional therapy that focuses on treating the cancer, but rather focuses on relieving their symptoms and quality of life. Regardless of which therapy a patient chooses, a thorough discussion with their treatment team should occur.

SETTING SHORT-TERM GOALS

Each patient's experience of cancer is unique and personal. It is perfectly natural for patients and their loved ones to experience a wide variety of emotions during diagnosis and treatment. Patients are faced with some of the most difficult decisions of their lives and these decisions are likely to get much more challenging when the cancer is in an advanced stage. Throughout the journey of cancer diagnosis and treatment patients should continually ask, "What are my overall goals?"

The following questions have helped many of our patients frame their goals:

- What makes life worth living?
- What are the most important things for me to achieve?
- What are my most important hopes?
- What are my biggest fears?
- What would I consider to be a fate worse than death?

These questions may seem overwhelming as we confront issues that most of us don't confront until we realize that our time to live might be shorter than we imagined. However, your answers to these questions will help you to know and understand what you, your loved ones, and healthcare providers should focus on to best support you through this process. For some patients their goals may be as simple as "I want to go on that 25th anniversary cruise we've had planned," or "I want to continue to work during my treatment." Goals may be related to your fears, for example, "Whatever we do, I don't want to be in pain." Your goals may overlap, "I want to be cured, but if I'm not, I want my family to be prepared." Your goals may seem contradictory to your doctors, nurses, and loved ones, but it is extremely important that your healthcare providers know your wishes.

CONSIDERATIONS AS YOU START PLANNING FOR YOUR FUTURE WITH CANCER

You and your loved ones are living with a new reality. It's not easy to consider your future, knowing, or NOT knowing how this will all end up. Having cancer means that plans will change and then probably change again. Patients need to consider the "what ifs." You and your oncologist have decided on a treatment plan, but, what if things don't go according to the plan? "Don't think about it!" or only considering the positive outcomes doesn't work with serious diseases like lung cancer. To protect yourself and your loved ones, you need to make decisions, and discuss them with your family and providers. To help you with these decisions you need to have honest and open discussions with your oncologist, even if the news may be bad, or not what you had hoped for. Ask questions. Don't be embarrassed to ask for explanations about terminology, stages of the cancer, if it has spread, and what it all means. You will need to have your treatment options explained in terms of the benefit to be achieved by the treatment versus the burden it may impose on your life. One way of looking at this is to ask your doctor, "In real terms (weeks, months or years) what can I realistically expect from this treatment in controlling or palliating my lung cancer? And how much will I be troubled or burdened by side effects of the treatment?"

Besides the medical treatment, other issues may need to be explored. These may include:

- How extensive is your medical insurance coverage? You may want to inquire if your insurance plans will allow supportive, palliative, or hospice care if you need it. Many states require insurance companies to cover the routine costs of treatment for patients on clinical trials, but others do not. If you are considering a clinical trial, especially early phase trials, be sure to discuss this with your insurance carrier before seeking to enroll in a study.

- If you are working, you will eventually need to discuss your condition with your employer. Consider what it would mean to you and your family if you had to decrease your work hours—especially if you are the sole source of income. Explore other benefits, such as disability insurance or family medical leave policies.

- You may also want to begin preparing for any legal issues that you or your family need to consider, such as wills, life insurance coverage, etc.

Finally, you will want to begin the task of advanced care planning. This can be done through medical advanced directives or living wills or using a document such as Five Wishes. Social workers, nurses, and physicians are prepared to help patients with these issues. These are very important documents to complete. You can start this discussion by going back to your goals and having an open and honest discussion with your doctor, family members, and loved ones who will be helping you make those very hard and emotional decisions concerning life support, should that ever be needed, and/or other aggressive treatments.

Common life supportive treatments include:

- *Cardiopulmonary resuscitation (CPR).* Doctors will usually frame this as "Do you want me to attempt to restart your heart and lungs if you are at the end of your life, if doing so would not change the course of your disease?" This would most likely require an admission to the intensive care unit and a prolonged hospitalization. You should talk with the doctor about chances of survival after resuscitation, and possible changes that may occur during and after resuscitation.

- *Intubation.* Many lung cancer patients face this decision at some point during the course of their disease. Intubation involves "connecting" your lungs to a breathing machine by inserting a tube through your mouth into the windpipe of your lungs. The tube is connected to a machine that breathes for you. Patients are usually sedated, and unable to speak or interact while on the breathing machine. Intubation may be suggested if you are having a lot of trouble breathing because of the cancer, pneumonia, or other medical condition. You should discuss this scenario with your doctor, and, as with CPR, what the realistic implications of advanced therapies are for patients with incurable diseases.

- *Eating and drinking, or artificial nutrition.* If you were unable to continue eating or drinking as a result of your cancer progression, would you want advanced nutritional support, such as feeding tubes or intravenous feeding (total parenteral nutrition, or TPN), to sustain your life? Patients and their loved ones often wrestle with this decision because stopping nutrition seems inhumane. Often, advanced nutritional support doesn't provide much benefit to patients with advanced cancer. Discuss these measures honestly with your trusted health professionals.

All too often, discussions concerning these important decisions occur during a time of crisis. This is extremely hard on loved ones, who are frightened and worried, and being pressured to make decisions quickly. The purpose of advanced directives is to avoid these difficult situations by making your wishes known in writing.

WHEN MIGHT I STOP TREATMENT?

Defining the moment in time when further aggressive cancer treatment offers little or no benefit is difficult for patients and their physicians. Life is fragile, precious, and unpredictable. Experienced oncologists and nurses can often identify patients for whom, in their opinion, further therapy is likely to offer very little benefit, only to be fooled. In our experience, patients who honestly listen to their own bodies and understand their personal, physical, and psychological response to their cancer can often provide the best insight. This period of illness is incredibly difficult for patients, their loved ones, and their treating healthcare professionals.

Establishing realistic, attainable goals and treatment plans with your doctor becomes more important as your cancer progresses. The medical literature tells us that most individuals with lung cancer want to have their pain, shortness of breath, and other symptoms relieved. Additionally our patients tell us that having a good quality of life and maintaining control over the final stages of their lives are also pivotal. With clear and deliberate planning, this can be achieved for most patients.

WHAT IS THE ROLE OF PALLIATIVE CARE AND HOSPICE?

PALLIATIVE CARE

The aim of palliative care is to relieve your suffering, improve your quality of life, and provide a source of support and comfort for your loved ones. Palliative care usually includes a team of doctors, nurses, social workers, pharmacists, and nutritionists with specific knowledge and skills to help patients manage pain, shortness of breath, fatigue, and other distressing physical symptoms. The palliative care team also provides psychosocial and spiritual support, and helps to coordinate an array of medical and social services. It is important for you to understand that palliative care can be offered simultaneously with other medical therapies that are directed at treating lung cancer. The intensity and range of palliative interventions will change and may increase as your cancer progresses. Palliative care providers attempt to remain sensitive to personal, cultural and religious values, beliefs, and practices. Palliative care professionals will also help to guide patients and their loved ones through the transitions and challenges involved in the end of life.

HOSPICE

Hospice care is a philosophy, or concept of care, that arose during the middle ages. A hospice at that time was a place where travelers, pilgrims, the sick, wounded, or dying could find rest and comfort. Today, hospice care is provided to patients who have a limited time to live (usually 6 months or less). While in a hospice program, you and your family will be the center of an approach to care in which life and living are affirmed, and dying is regarded as a normal process.

Hospice emphasizes care, comfort, and quality of life by managing pain and other distressing symptoms. A team of providers including doctors, nurses, home health aides, social workers, chaplains, counselors, and trained volunteers will be assigned to you and your family. The hospice team develops a care plan that meets your individual needs by working together and focusing on physical symptoms, and offering emotional and spiritual support.

In the United States, most hospice care is provided in your home but other options for care are available, depending on your symptoms or if your family needs respite (a rest) for a short period of time. By being there for you and your family, the hospice team provides personalized care to prepare you and your family for your eventual dying and death. Hospice care continues after death, by offering bereavement/grief support to those family members and loved ones who are in need of support.

SUMMARY

The goal of treatment for metastatic lung cancer is cancer control and the palliation of symptoms produced by advanced cancer. Treatment that is directed at lessening the side effects from treatment and improvement of quality of life are other important goals of care.

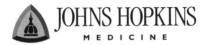

CHAPTER 10

LUNG CANCER IN OLDER ADULTS

GARY R. SHAPIRO, MD

L ung cancer is the leading cause of cancer deaths in the world, and, with a median age of diagnosis at 70 years, it is closely linked with the elderly. As we live longer, the number of men and women with lung cancer will increase dramatically. In the next 25 years, the number of people who are 65 years of age and older will double, and the largest increases in cancer incidence will occur in those older than 80 years of age.

Older adults with cancer often have other chronic health problems, and may be taking multiple medications that can affect their cancer treatment plan. Prejudice, misunderstanding, and limited access to clinical trials often prevent older patients from getting the timely cancer treatment that they need.

When a lung cancer is found in the elderly it is too often ignored or under treated. Older individuals have less surgery and less radiation therapy. They do not always get appropriate adjuvant chemotherapy therapy, and their metastatic lung cancer is often left untreated. As a result, older adults often have much worse outcomes than younger patients.

WHY IS THERE MORE CANCER IN OLDER PEOPLE?

The organs in our body are made up of cells, which divide and multiply as the body needs them. Cancer develops when cells in a part of the body grow out of control. The body has a number of ways of repairing damaged control mechanisms, but as we get older, these methods do not work as well. Although our healthier lifestyles have allowed us to avoid death from infection, heart attack, and stroke, we may now live long enough for a cancer to develop. People who live longer have increased exposure to cancer-causing agents (carcinogens) in the environment, like tobacco, asbestos, and other workplace substances. Aging decreases the body's ability to protect us from carcinogens and to repair cells that are damaged by these and other processes.

LUNG CANCER IS DIFFERENT IN OLDER PEOPLE

Older people are more likely to present with potentially curable early stage lung cancer than their younger counterparts. Part of the reason for this stage-to-age trend is a change in lung cancer subtypes (see Table 1) with age. There are twice as many squamous cell carcinomas in 80-year-olds than in 40-year-olds (with a proportionate decrease in adenocarcinoma and SCLC). Age itself may play more of a role in the course of SCLC than it does in NSCLC; those younger than 65 do better than those older than 65.

DECISION MAKING: 7 PRACTICAL STEPS

1. GET A DIAGNOSIS

Although most lung masses in older people are malignant, many are granulomas, or benign collections of inflammatory or scar tissue. Some are due to infections or other treatable nonmalignant diseases. Not all malignant lung nodules are due to lung cancer, and your prognosis and treatment options may be vastly different depending upon the kind of cancer that you have.

Even among lung cancers, there is a world of difference between a SCLC and a NSCLC. SCLC grows very fast; NSCLC grows much slower. SCLC usually responds to chemotherapy within weeks; NSCLC takes longer and is more likely to be resistant to systemic therapy. SCLC is always treated with chemotherapy, while the slower growing non-small cell type is best treated with surgery in its early stage.

A diagnosis helps you and your family to understand what to expect and how to prepare for the future, even if you cannot get curative treatment. Knowing the diagnosis also helps your doctor to better treat your symptoms. Many people find not knowing very hard, and are relieved when they finally have an explanation for their symptoms. Sometimes a frail patient is obviously dying, and diagnostic studies can be an additional burden. In such cases, it may be quite reasonable to focus on symptom relief (palliation) without knowing the details of the diagnosis.

2. KNOW THE CANCER'S STAGE

The cancer's stage defines your prognosis and treatment options. No one can make informed decisions without it. Just as there may be times when the burdens of diagnostic studies may be too great, it may also be appropriate to do without full staging in very frail, dying patient. As with younger patients, stage is determined by the size of the tumor, the presence or absence of cancer in chest lymph nodes or its spread (metastasis) to other organs. When doctors combine this information with information regarding your cancer's subtype, they can predict what impact, if any, your lung cancer is likely to have on your life expectancy and quality of life.

3. KNOW YOUR LIFE EXPECTANCY

Anti-cancer treatment should be considered if you are likely to live long enough to experience symptoms or premature death from lung cancer. If your life expectancy is so short that the cancer will not significantly affect it, there may be no reason to treat your cancer. However, chronological age should not be the only thing that decides how your cancer should, or should not, be treated. Despite advanced age, people who are relatively well often have a life expectancy that is longer than their life expectancy with lung cancer. The average 70-year-old woman is likely to live another 16 years, and the average 70-year-old man another 12 years. A similar 85-year-old can expect to live an additional 5 to 6 years, and remain independent for most of that time. Even an unhealthy 75-year-old man or woman probably will live 5 to 6 more years, long enough to suffer symptoms and early death from recurrent lung cancer.

4. UNDERSTAND THE GOALS

The Goals of Treatment

It is important to be clear whether the goal of treatment is cure (surgery and adjuvant chemotherapy for early stage NSCLC, or chemotherapy for limited stage SCLC) or palliation (treatment for incurable advanced metastatic lung cancer). If the goal is palliation, you need to understand if the treatment plan will extend your life, control your symptoms, or both. It is also important to know how likely is it to achieve these goals, and how long you will enjoy the benefits of palliation.

When the goal of treatment is palliation, chemotherapy should never be administered without defined endpoints and timelines. It should be clear to everyone what "counts" as success, how it will be determined (for example, a symptom controlled or a smaller mass on CT scan), and when. You and your family should understand what your options are at each step, and how likely each is to meet your goals. If this is not clear, ask your doctor to explain it in words that you understand.

The Goals of the Patient

In addition to the traditional goals of tumor response, increased survival, and symptom control, older cancer patients often have goals related to quality of life. These may include physical and intellectual independence, spending quality time with your family, taking trips, staying out of the hospital, or even economic stability. At times, palliative care or hospice may meet these goals better than active anticancer treatment. In addition to the medical team, older patients often turn to family, friends and clergy to help guide them.

5. DETERMINE IF YOU ARE FIT OR FRAIL

Deciding how to treat cancer in someone who is older requires a thorough understanding of his or her general health and social situation. Decisions about cancer treatment should never focus on age alone.

Age is Not a Number

Your actual age has limited influence on how cancer will respond to therapy or its prognosis. Biological and other changes associated with aging are more reliable in estimating an individual's vigor, life expectancy, or the risk of treatment complications. These changes include malnutrition, loss of muscle mass and strength, depression, dementia, falls, social isolation, and the ability to accomplish daily activities such as dressing, bathing, eating, shopping, housekeeping, and managing one's finances or medication.

Chronic Illnesses

Older cancer patients are likely to have chronic illnesses (comorbidity) that affect their life expectancy; the more that you have, the greater the effect. This effect has very little impact on the behavior of the cancer itself, but studies do show that comorbidity has a major impact on treatment outcome and its side effects.

6. BALANCE BENEFITS AND HARMS

Fit, older lung cancer patients respond to treatment similarly to their younger counterparts. However, a word of caution is in order. Until recently, few studies included older individuals, and it may not be appropriate to apply these findings to the diverse group of older cancer patients.

The side effects of cancer treatment are never less in the elderly. In addition to the standard side effects, there are significant age-related toxicities to consider. Though most of these are more a function of frailty than chronological age, even the fittest senior cannot avoid the physical effects of aging. In addition to the changes in fat and muscle that you see in the mirror, there are age-related changes in your kidney, liver, and digestive (gastrointestinal) function. These changes affect how your body absorbs and metabolizes anticancer drugs and other medicines. The average older man or woman takes many different medicines to control health issues like high blood pressure, high cholesterol, osteoporosis, diabetes, and arthritis. This polypharmacy can cause undesirable side effects because the many drugs interact with each other and the anticancer medications.

7. GET INVOLVED

Healthcare providers and family members often underestimate the physical and mental abilities of older people and their willingness to face chronic and life-threatening conditions. Studies clearly show that older patients want detailed and easily-understood information about potential treatments and alternatives. Patients and families may consider cancer untreatable in the aged, and not understand the possibilities offered by treatment.

While patients with dementia pose a unique challenge, they are frequently capable of participating in goal setting and simple discussions about treatment side effects and logistics. Caring family members and friends are often able to share the patient's life story so that healthcare workers can work with them to make decisions consistent with the patient's values and desires. This of course is no substitute for a well thought out and properly executed living will or healthcare proxy.

While it is hard to face the possibility of life-threatening events at any age, it is always better to be prepared and to put your affairs in order. In addition to estate planning and wills, it is critical that you outline your wishes regarding medical care at the end of life, and make legal provisions for someone to make those decisions if you are unable to make them for yourself.

TREATING LUNG CANCER

YOU NEED A TEAM

Cancer care changes rapidly, and it is hard for the generalist to keep up to date, so referral to a specialist is essential. The needs of an older cancer patient often extend beyond the doctor's office and the traditional services provided by visiting nurses. These needs may include transportation; nutrition; and emotional, financial, physical, or spiritual support. When an older person with lung cancer is the primary caregiver for a frail or ill spouse, grandchildren, or other family members, special attention is necessary to provide for their needs as well. Older cancer patients cared for in geriatric oncology programs benefit from multidisciplinary teams of oncologists, geriatricians, psychiatrists, pharmacists, physiatrists, social workers, nurses, clergy, and dieticians, all working together as a team to identify and manage the stressors that can limit effective cancer treatment.

TREATING NSCLC

SURGERY

Though lung cancer surgery is often complex, it is the standard of care for most early stage NSCLCs (see Chapter 3), regardless of age. It is as effective in elderly patients as in younger patients, but it does have a somewhat higher rate of complications in older individuals who have other medical problems (comorbidities). Like other treatment options, surgery in some older individuals may involve risks related to decreases in body organ function (especially heart and lung), and it is essential that the surgeon and anesthetist work closely with your primary care physician or a consultant to fully assess and treat these problems before, during, and after the operation. Radiofrequency ablation (see pages 53–54) may be an option for frail individuals, or those with a very high surgical risk, who have small stage I tumors.

RADIATION THERAPY

Radiation therapy is rarely the treatment of choice for early stage (I and II) cancer of the lung. In these stages, it is reserved for the very frail or those at great risk from surgery. Doctors do use it, often in combination with chemotherapy, as an essential part of the treatment for inoperable locally advanced stage III NSCLC (see Chapter 3). It is just as effective in older patients as it is in younger patients.

Radiation therapy can cause swallowing problems and pain due to esophagitis (inflammation and irritation of the esophagus). Although temporary and treatable, these symptoms are usually more problematic in older patients who are already at risk for dehydration and malnutrition. Dehydration, weight loss, and electrolyte disturbances are preventable with careful monitoring.

Radiation therapy usually provides excellent symptom relief (palliation) in metastatic and other incurable situations. It is particularly effective in treating pain caused by lung cancer metastases to the bone. A short course of radiation therapy often allows patients with advanced cancer to lower (or even eliminate) their dose of narcotic pain relievers. Although these medicines do an excellent job of controlling pain, they often cause confusion, falls, and constipation in older patients. Thus, even hospice patients suffering from localized metastatic bone pain should consider the option of palliative radiation therapy. It also provides excellent palliation of symptoms due to brain metastases.

The fatigue that usually accompanies radiation therapy can be quite profound in the elderly, even in those who are fit. Often the logistical details (like daily travel to the hospital for several weeks of treatment) are the hardest for older people. It is important that you discuss these potential problems with your family and social worker, prior to starting radiation therapy.

CHEMOTHERAPY

Chemotherapy is an essential part of the treatment (see Chapter 3) of all stages of SCLC, and inoperable NSCLC that has not metastasized (stage III). In combination with radiation therapy, it often gives NSCLC patients years of life that they would not otherwise have. It is an important adjunct to surgery in those whose NSCLC has been completely removed but who are at risk for recurrence (stages II & IIIA). It is also a useful and effective option for controlling symptoms and increasing longevity in non-frail seniors with advanced metastatic NSCLC.

Nonfrail older cancer patients respond to chemotherapy similarly to their younger counterparts. Reducing the dose of chemotherapy (or radiation therapy) based purely on chronological age may seriously affect the effectiveness of treatment. On the other hand, older patients may need lower doses if they have reduced kidney or liver function.

Managing chemotherapy-associated toxicity with appropriate supportive care is crucial in the elderly population to give them the best chance of cure and survival or to provide the best palliation.

Older lung cancer patients have higher rates of fatigue, mouth sores (mucositis), diarrhea, neutropenia (low white blood cell count that can increase the risk of infection), thrombocytopenia (low platelet blood count that can cause bleeding), and kidney (nephrotoxicity) side effects. Severe side effects are more common in Platinol-AQ–based chemotherapy programs than those that use other drugs like Paraplatin. Most targeted therapy like Tarceva is as effective and well tolerated in the elderly as it is in younger patients. However, there does appear to be an increased risk of blood clots and other vascular problems with Avastin, especially in those with hypertension or cardiovascular problems. Avastin can also cause gastrointestinal side effects (including obstruction and perforation), which are especially troublesome in older patients who are predisposed to constipation.

Though the side effects of cancer treatment are never less burdensome in the elderly, they can be managed by oncologists, especially geriatric oncologists, who work in teams with others who specialize in the care of the elderly. With appropriate care, healthy older patients do just as well with chemotherapy as younger patients. Advances in supportive care (antinausea medicines and blood cell growth factors) have significantly decreased the side effects of chemotherapy, and improved safety and the quality of life of individuals with lung cancer. Nonetheless, there is risk, especially if the patient is frail. The presence of severe comorbidities, age-related frailty or underlying severe psychosocial problems may be obstacles for highly intensive treatment plans.

Such patients may benefit from less complicated or potentially less toxic treatment plans.

When choosing a palliative chemotherapy regimen, preference should be given to chemotherapeutic drugs with safer profiles, such as Gemzar, Navelbine, or weekly taxane regimens. Single agent therapy is less toxic, and probably just as effective as combination chemotherapy in metastatic lung cancer.

TREATING SCLC

As in younger patients, chemotherapy is used to treat all stages of SCLC. There is no role for surgery. Radiation to the chest and brain is added to chemotherapy for those with limited stage disease. It is also used to palliate symptoms of advanced SCLC, especially bone and brain metastases. The side effects of radiation therapy and chemotherapy for older individuals with SCLC are no different than those discussed for NSCLC in the section above.

Unlike NSCLC, chronological age does predict for response to chemotherapy in SCLC. SCLC tends to be more resistant to treatment in those over 65 years old. Nevertheless, intensive chemotherapy offers better hope for palliation of advanced SCLC and its symptoms than it does for NSCLC. Metastatic NSCLC usually grows at a plodding pace over many months, with modest responses to chemotherapy that need to be carefully balanced against quality of life concerns. In contrast, SCLC grows rapidly over several weeks, usually responding dramatically to chemotherapy within a very short period of time, sometimes even several days. Although chemotherapy for SCLC can be tough, there is little doubt that it is the best way to control symptoms in all but the most frail man or woman with SCLC.

COMMON TREATMENT COMPLICATIONS IN
THE ELDERLY

Anemia (low red blood cell count) is common in the elderly, especially the frail elderly. It decreases the effectiveness of chemotherapy, and often causes fatigue, falls, cognitive decline (for example, dementia, disorientation, or confusion), and heart problems. Therefore, it is essential that anemia be recognized and corrected with red blood cell transfusions or the appropriate use of erythropoiesis-stimulating agents like Procrit or Epogen (epoetin) or Aranesp (darbepoetin).

Myelosuppression (low white blood cell count) is also common in older patients getting chemotherapy or radiation therapy. Older patients with myelosuppression develop life-threatening infections more often than younger patients, and they may need to be treated in the hospital for many days. The liberal use of granulopoietic growth factors (or G-CSF, including Neupogen [filgrastim] and Neulasta [pegfilgrastim]) decreases the risk of infection, and makes it possible for older patients to receive full doses of potentially curable adjuvant chemotherapy.

Mucositis (mouth sores), esophagitis (inflammation of the esophagus), and diarrhea can cause severe dehydration in older patients, who often are already dehydrated due to inadequate fluid intake and diuretics ("water pills" taken for high blood pressure or heart failure). Careful monitoring and the liberal use of antidiarrheal agents (Imodium) and oral and intravenous fluids are essential components of the management of older cancer patients, especially those receiving lung radiation or Gemzar, or both.

Kidney function declines as we age. Some of the medicines that older patients take to treat both their cancer-related (for example, Platinol-AQ, Paraplatin, and NSAIDs) and noncancer-related problems might make this worse. The dehydration that often accompanies cancer and its treatment can put additional stress on the kidneys. Fortunately, it is often possible to minimize these effects by carefully selecting and dosing appropriate drugs, managing polypharmacy, and preventing dehydration.

Neurotoxicity and cognitive effects (chemo-brain) can be profoundly debilitating in patients who are already cognitively impaired (demented, disoriented, confused, etc.). Elderly patients with a history of falling, hearing loss, or peripheral neuropathy (for example, nerve damage from diabetes) have decreased energy, and are highly vulnerable to neurotoxic chemotherapy like the taxanes or platinum compounds. Many of the medicines used to control nausea (antiemetics) or decrease the side effects of certain chemotherapeutic agents are also potential neurotoxins. These include Decadron (psychosis and agitation), Zantac (agitation), Benadryl, and some of the antiemetics (sedation). Whole brain radiation therapy can also make underlying cognitive impairment worse.

Fatigue is a near universal complaint of older cancer patients. It is particularly a problem for those who are socially isolated or depend upon others to help them with activities of daily living. It is not necessarily related to depression, but can be. Depression is quite common in the elderly. In contrast to younger patients who often respond to a cancer diagnosis with anxiety, depression is the more common disorder in older cancer patients. With proper support and medical attention, many of these patients can safely receive anticancer treatment.

Heart problems increase with age, and it is no surprise that older cancer patients have an increased risk of cardiac complications from intensive surgery, radiation, and chemotherapy. Patients treated with Platinol-AQ chemotherapy require large amounts of intravenous fluid hydration. This can cause congestive heart failure in patients with heart problems; they need careful monitoring.

CHAPTER 11

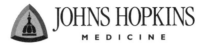

JOHNS HOPKINS
M E D I C I N E

TRUSTED RESOURCES—FINDING ADDITIONAL INFORMATION ABOUT LUNG CANCER AND ITS TREATMENT

TERESA SEEGER, CRNP; AND JULIE R. BRAHMER, MD

L ack of information about lung cancer is not a problem. In fact, the reverse is true. There are multiple sources of varying quality. As you pursue your own search for information, remember to be a critical consumer. We believe the following are good sources of information, but remember, you and your loved one are unique. No organization or publication can ever replace the judgment of your trusted physicians and healthcare professionals. Be informed and ask lots of questions!

- *Consider the source.* This is especially true of Web sites. Anyone can post anything on the web. None of it has to be accurate. Look for sites and information from the government, national cancer and lung organizations, and hospitals. Most sites have a link explaining the goals of the organization.

- *Is the information based on research?* The most reliable information comes from clinical trials.

- *Opinions/recommendations may vary between sources.* Treating cancer can be art as well as science. Frequently there is no one "right" answer.

- *Beware of the mass media.* Headlines often do not tell the entire picture.

- *What works for one may not work for anyone else.* Talking to other cancer patients can be an excellent source of information but remember that every cancer is different and every person is different.

- *Do not act on what you read without asking your healthcare provider.* The information may not apply to your situation, but the recommendation could be harmful rather than helpful to you.

LUNG CANCER SPECIFIC

American Lung Association
The American Lung Association is a nonprofit organization that "fights" lung disease in all its forms, with special emphasis on asthma, tobacco control, and air quality.

800-LUNG-USA
http://www.lungusa.org
Lung Cancer—Making Treatment Decisions
http://www.lungusa.org/lung-disease/lung-cancer/living-with-lung-cancer/making-treatment-decisions/

Lung Cancer Alliance

Lung Cancer Information Line, (800) 298-2436
http://www.lungcanceralliance.org

This is a national non-profit organization dedicated solely to patient support and advocacy for people living with lung cancer and those at risk for the disease.

LungCancer.org

(800) 813-HOPE (4673)
http://www.lungcancer.org

This is a program of Cancer*Care*, a national nonprofit organization that provides free, professional support services to anyone affected by cancer.

National Lung Cancer Partnership

(608) 233-7905
http://www.NationalLungCancerPartnership.org

This is a group of leading doctors, researchers, patient advocates, and lung cancer survivors who are working together to improve treatments for lung cancer patients. The group is dedicated to raising public awareness of the disease and generating funding for lung cancer research.

GENERAL CANCER

American Cancer Society

(800) ACS-2345
http://www.cancer.org

General cancer information Web site.

Cancer.net

> http://www.cancer.net
> (888) 651-3038

Oncologist-approved information from the American Society of Clinical Oncologists on more than 120 types of cancer and cancer-related syndromes.

Cancer*Care*

> http://www.cancercare.org
> (800) 813-HOPE (4673)

Cancer*Care* is a national nonprofit organization that provides free, professional support services for anyone affected by cancer.

MD Anderson Cancer Center

> http://www.mdanderson.org/

The Anderson Network through the MD Anderson Cancer Center is a great patient-to-patient support network that can be accessed over the phone.

MedlinePlus

> http://www.medlineplus.gov

Information from the US National Library of Medicine and the NIH.

National Cancer Institute

> Cancer Information Service, (800) 4-CANCER
> (422-6237)
> http://www.cancer.gov
> Lung Cancer—http://www.cancer.gov/cancertopics/types/lung

Provides information about treatment, including surgery, chemotherapy, radiation therapy, immunotherapy, and vaccine therapy.

Booklets: The NCI has many booklets available on a wide variety of topics, including the following:

- Chemotherapy & You

- Coping With Advanced Cancer

- Eating Hints for Cancer Patients

- Get Relief from Cancer Pain

- Radiotherapy & You

- Taking Time: Support for People with Cancer

- What You Need to Know about Lung Cancer

- When Cancer Returns

- When Someone in Your Family Has Cancer

National Coalition for Cancer Survivorship (NCCS)

(877) NCCS-YES (622-7937)
http://www.canceradvocacy.org

NCCS, a helpful organization for cancer survivors, publishes The Cancer Survival Toolbox, which is a free, self-learning audio program developed by cancer organizations to help people develop important skills to meet and understand the challenges of their cancer diagnosis. The toolbox contains a set of basic skills to help navigate diagnosis, and special topics on key issues faced by people with cancer. You can order a free CD version of the program online or by phone.

National Comprehensive Cancer Network (NCCN)

(215) 690-0300

http://www.nccn.com/

NCCN is an alliance of 21 of the world's leading cancer centers, working together to develop treatment guidelines for most cancers, and dedicated to research that improves the quality, effectiveness, and efficiency of cancer care.

Oncolink

(215) 349-8895

http://www.oncolink.com

University of Pennsylvania Abramson Cancer Center site with comprehensive information about specific cancer types, updates on cancer treatments, and news about research advances. The site updates the information every day and provides information at various levels, from introductory to in-depth.

MEDICATION

Many of the pharmaceutical companies have brochures and Web sites dedicated to their drugs. Ask your healthcare provider.

NUTRITION

American Institute for Cancer Research

(800) 843-8114

http://www.aicr.org

Cancer charity that fosters research on diet and cancer prevention, interprets the evidence, and educates the public about the results.

RADIATION THERAPY

American Society for Radiation Oncology

(703) 502-1550

http://www.astro.org/

This Web site explains how radiation therapy is used to safely and effectively treat cancer.

REFERENCE

Caring Connection

http://www.caringinfo.org/stateaddownload

Caring Connection raises financial support for human service agencies by helping donors directly support local organizations they know and trust.

Complementary and Alternative Medicine

(888) 644-6226

http://nccam.nih.gov

Research-based information on treatments and conditions from the NIH.

Five Wishes

http://www.agingwithdignity.org/five-wishes.php

Five Wishes helps you express how you want to be treated if you are seriously ill and unable to speak for yourself. It deals with all of a person's needs.

Lab Tests Online

http://www.labtestsonline.org

Lab Tests Online is the product of collaboration among professional societies representing the clinical laboratory community. Lab Tests Online has been designed to help better understand many clinical lab tests.

Medical Dictionary

http://www.mondofacto.com/facts/dictionary?

This Web site offers a searchable dictionary of terms from medicine, science, and technology.

Surgeon General

http://www.surgeongeneral.gov/tobacco

The Office of the Surgeon General (OSG), under the direction of the Surgeon General, oversees the operations of the 6,000-member Commissioned Corps of the U.S. Public Service. The Office provides the best scientific information available on how to improve American's health and reduce the risk of illness and injury.

SIDE EFFECTS

Oncology Nurses Society

(866) 257-4ONS (257-4667)
http://www.cancersymptoms.org

Web site designed for patients and caregivers to provide information on learning about and managing each of 10 most common cancer treatment-related symptoms.

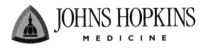

JOHNS HOPKINS
M E D I C I N E

INFORMATION ABOUT
JOHNS HOPKINS

The Johns Hopkins Thoracic Oncology Program
Lung Cancer is part of the Upper Aerodigestive
Cancer Program
Appointment Line: (410) 955-8893

The goal of the Johns Hopkins Thoracic Oncology Program
is to reduce the morbidity and mortality of lung cancer. We
provide comprehensive lung cancer services including prevention, screening, diagnosis, treatment, and access to the
latest and most promising therapies. Our thoracic oncology team has experience in multiple disciplines allowing
us to provide our patients with the highest quality and compassionate care. Our program also promotes research that
develops innovative and improved methods for diagnosing
and treating the disease.

Sidney Kimmel Comprehensive Cancer Center at Johns Hopkins
http://www.hopkinskimmelcancercenter.org

Since its inception in 1973, the Sidney Kimmel Comprehensive Cancer Center at Johns Hopkins has been dedicated to better understanding human cancers and finding more effective treatments. One of only forty cancer centers in the country designated by the National Cancer Institute (http://www.cancer.gov) as a Comprehensive Cancer Center, the Johns Hopkins Kimmel Cancer Center has active programs in clinical research, laboratory research, education, community outreach, and prevention and control, and is the only Comprehensive Cancer Center in the state of Maryland.

About Johns Hopkins Medicine
http://www.hopkinsmedicine.org

Johns Hopkins Medicine unites physicians and scientists of the Johns Hopkins University School of Medicine with the organizations, health professionals, and facilities of the Johns Hopkins Health System. Its mission is to improve the health of the community and the world by setting the standard of excellence in medical education, research, and clinical care. Diverse and inclusive, Johns Hopkins Medicine has provided international leadership in the education of physicians and medical scientists in biomedical research and in the application of medical knowledge to sustain health since The Johns Hopkins Hospital opened in 1889.

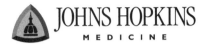

FURTHER READING

100 Questions & Answers About How to Quit Smoking, Charles Herrick, MD; Charlotte Herrick, RN, PhD; and Marianne Mitchell, ARNP; Jones and Bartlett Publishers, 2010.

100 Questions & Answers About Lung Cancer, Second Edition, Karen Parles, MLS; Joan H. Schiller, MD; and Amy Cipau; Jones and Bartlett Publishers, 2010.

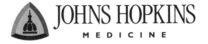

GLOSSARY

Adenocarcinoma: A type of non-small cell lung cancer; a malignant tumor that arises from glandular tissue.

Adjuvant therapy: Treatment given after the primary treatment to increase the chances of a cure, and treatment to prevent the cancer from recurring.

Alveoli: Tiny air sacs that compose the lungs.

Angiogenesis: The formation of new blood vessels that allows tumors to grow.

Angiogenesis inhibitors: Drugs that prevent the formation of new blood vessels.

Antiemetics: Antinausea medications.

Asymptomatic: Without symptoms.

Bilateral: Both sides.

Biopsy: A procedure in which cells are collected for microscopic examination.

Bone scan: An X-ray that looks for signs of metastasis.

Brachytherapy: A form of internal radiation therapy that involves placing "seeds" of radioactive material near or in the tumor.

Bronchioloalveolar carcinoma (BAC): A type of adenocarcinoma.

Bronchoscopy: A procedure that involves inserting a long, narrow, flexible tube (bronchoscope) through the nose down into the lungs. Needles can be inserted through the bronchoscope to obtain biopsy samples.

Bronchus: One of the large air tubes.

Cancer: The presence of malignant cells.

Carcinogen: Cancer-causing substance.

Carcinomas: Cancers that form in the surface cells of different tissues.

Cells: Basic elements of tissues; the appearance and composition of individual cells are unique to the tissue they compose.

Chemo brain: Difficulty with cognitive functioning as a side effect of receiving chemotherapy.

Chemotherapy: The use of chemical agents (drugs) to systemically treat cancer.

Clinical trial: A study of a drug or treatment with a large group testing the treatment.

Comorbidity: A disease or disorder someone already has prior to a new diagnosis. Examples include diabetes, heart disease, and a previous history of blood clots.

Complementary therapy: Medicines used in conjunction with standard therapies.

CT (computed tomography) scan: Computerized series of X-rays that create a detailed cross-sectional image of the body.

Drain: A small tube inserted into a wound cavity to collect fluid.

Fibrosis: Scarring of the lung.

Field: The treatment site.

Healthcare proxy: A document that permits a designated person to make decisions regarding your medical treatment when you are unable to do so.

Hilar lymph nodes: Lymph nodes located in the region where the bronchus meets the lung.

Incidence: The number of times a disease occurs within a population of people.

Intravenous: In the vein.

Invasive cancer: Cancer that breaks through normal lung tissue barriers and invades surrounding areas.

Large cell carcinoma: A type of non-small cell lung cancer.

Living will: A document that outlines what care you want in the event that you become unable to communicate due to coma or heavy sedation.

Lobectomy: Surgical removal of a lobe of the lung.

Lymph: Fluid carried through the body by the lymphatic system, composed primarily of white blood cells and diluted plasma.

Lymph nodes: Tissues in the lymphatic system that filter lymph fluid and help the immune system fight disease.

Lymphatic system: A collection of vessels with the principle functions of transporting digested fat from the intestine to the bloodstream, removing and destroying toxins from tissues, and resisting the spread of disease throughout the body.

Lymphedema: A condition in which lymph fluid collects in tissues following the removal of or damage to lymph nodes during surgery, causing the limb or area of the body affected to swell.

Main stem bronchi: The two main breathing tubes (right main stem bronchus and left main stem bronchus) that branch off the trachea.

Malignant: Cancerous; growing rapidly and out of control.

Mediastinal lymph nodes: Lymph nodes located in the mediastinum, the area between the lungs.

Mediastinoscopy: A surgical procedure by which lymph nodes can be removed for microscopic examination.

Metastasis, metastasize: The spread of cancer to other organ sites.

Mini-thoracotomy: A type of minimally invasive chest surgery.

Mortality: The statistical calculation of death rates due to a specific disease within a population.

Mutated: Altered.

Neoadjuvant therapy: Therapy given before the primary therapy; for example, neoadjuvant chemotherapy, which is sometimes given prior to surgery.

Neovascularization: Formation of new blood vessels that allows tumors to grow.

Neutropenia: A condition of an abnormally low number of a particular type of white blood cell called a neutrophil. White blood cells (leukocytes) are cells in the blood that play an important part in fighting off infection.

Noninvasive cancer: Cancer confined to its tissue point of origin and not found in surrounding tissue.

Non-small cell lung cancer (NSCLC): A type of lung cancer that includes adenocarcinoma, squamous cell carcinoma, and large cell carcinoma.

Oncologist: A cancer specialist who helps determine treatment choices.

Palliative care: Care to relieve the symptoms of cancer and to keep the best quality of life for as long as possible without seeking to cure cancer.

Pancoast tumor (superior sulcus tumor): A tumor occurring near the top of the lungs that may cause shoulder pain or weakness, or a group of symptoms including a droopy eyelid, dry eyes, and lack of sweating on the face.

Parietal pleura: A membrane lining the chest wall.

Pathologist: A specialist trained to distinguish normal from abnormal cells.

Peripheral neuropathy: Tingling, numbness, or burning sensation in hands, feet, or legs caused by damage to peripheral nerves by a tumor or by chemotherapy or radiation.

PET (positron emission tomography) scan: A nuclear medicine imaging test that measures metabolism; can differentiate between healthy and abnormal tissue.

Phases: A series of steps followed in clinical trials.

Placebo: An inert treatment (such as sugar pills) given in clinical trials to determine how much of a medicine's value is psychological.

Pleura: A membrane surrounding the lung (visceral pleura) and lining the chest wall (parietal pleura).

Pleural effusion: Accumulation of fluid between the outside of the lung and the inside of the chest wall.

Pleural space: The area between the outside of the lung and the inside of the chest wall.

Pleurodesis: A procedure to prevent recurrence of pleural effusion by draining the fluid and inserting medication into the pleural space.

Pneumonectomy: Surgical removal of the entire lung.

Pneumonia: An inflammatory infection of the lung.

Pneumonitis: Irritation of the lungs.

Post traumatic stress disorder: Emotional disorder resulting in a high level of anxiety and sometimes depression caused by a traumatic event in the past.

Primary care doctor: Regular physician who gives medical check-ups.

Prognosis: An estimation of the likely outcome of an illness based upon the patient's current status and the available treatments.

Protocol: The research plan for how long a drug is given and to whom it is given.

Pulmonary embolism (PE): A blood clot that travels to the lungs causing full or partial blockage of one or both pulmonary arteries.

Pulmonary function tests (PFTs): A group of breathing tests used to determine lung health.

Pulmonologist: A physician who specializes in the diagnosis and treatment of lung diseases.

Radiation oncologist: A cancer specialist who determines the amount of radiation therapy required.

Radiation therapy: Use of high-energy X-rays to kill cancer cells and shrink tumors.

Radiologist: A physician specializing in the treatment of disease using radiation therapy.

Red blood cells: Cells in the blood whose primary function is to carry oxygen to tissues.

Respiratory depression: Slowing of breathing.

Risk factors: Any factors that contribute to an increased possibility of getting cancer.

Second-line treatment: Treatment method(s) used following an initial treatment that either does not stop cancer progression or stops it only temporarily.

Small cell carcinoma: A type of lung cancer that differs in appearance and behavior from non-small cell lung cancers (adenocarcinoma, squamous cell carcinoma, large cell carcinoma).

Small cell lung cancer (SCLC): Refers to small cell carcinoma, as opposed to non-small cell lung cancers (adenocarcinoma, squamous cell carcinoma, large cell carcinoma).

Solvent: A substance, often a liquid, in which other substances are dissolved.

Sputum: Mucus and other secretions produced by the lungs.

Squamous cell carcinoma: A type of non-small cell lung cancer.

Stage: A numerical determination of how far the cancer has progressed.

Superior vena cava syndrome (SVCS): A collection of symptoms that may include swelling in the neck, shoulders, and arms caused by a lung tumor pressing on the superior vena cava, one of the large vessels leading into the heart.

Surgical oncologist: A specialist trained in surgical removal of cancerous tumors.

Systemic treatment: A treatment that affects the whole body (the patient's whole system).

Targeted therapy: Treatment that targets specific molecules involved in carcinogenesis or tumor growth.

Thoracentesis: A procedure that uses a needle to remove fluid from the space between the lung and the chest wall.

Thoracic surgeon: A surgeon who specializes in performing chest surgery.

Thoracotomy: A common type of lung surgery that requires a large incision to provide access to the lungs.

Trachea: Breathing tube (airway) leading from the larynx to the lungs.

Transthoracic (percutaneous) biopsy: A biopsy obtained by inserting a needle through the skin and chest wall into the tumor.

Tumor: Mass or lump of extra tissue.

Visceral pleura: A membrane surrounding the lung.

Wedge resection: Surgical removal of the tumor and a small amount of lung tissue surrounding the tumor.

White blood cells: A type of blood cell that fights infection.

X-ray: High-energy radiation used to image the body.

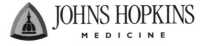

INDEX